'Through her blogs Nora expre[...] her deep understanding of the five [...] with humility, passion and the insigh[...] [...]on's guardian element. Nora never claims infallibility; instead she shares her uncertainties and mistakes so that we too may learn, as she has. Her best book yet, it offers much food for thought.'

– ROB RANSOME, *former Vice-Principal at SOFEA,*
Five Element Acupuncturist and Counsellor

'This collection conveys Nora Franglen's deep understanding of the five elements and the world of acupuncture. Nora's journey as a practitioner, teacher (and Londoner!), and her views on life and the world at large make for a heart-warming and thought-provoking read. Her writings bring the elements into my everyday life, helping me understand myself and others better.'

– SUJATA VARADARAJAN, *Scientist, Writer,*
sujatavaradarajan.blogspot.in

'The experience of reading Nora Franglen's latest book is akin to sitting with her in one of her beloved London cafés, listening to her as she holds forth on the Five Elements. Nora envelops the reader in the abundant joy she brings to her ever-evolving work as a "practical acupuncturist" astutely and with refreshingly frank introspection. This book is an invaluable, inspiring resource for anyone with an interest in the practice and life of a Five Element acupuncturist and teacher.'

– KERSTIN LEHR, *Acupuncture Intern, The*
Acupuncture Academy, Leamington Spa, UK

'If you are interested in making sense of our demanding, draining and complex world, *On Being a Five Element Acupuncturist* offers a precious window into it. With a lifetime's practice of seeing and working with the most subtle energies of the body, Nora's hard-earned wisdom and thought-provoking observations offer a rarely found depth of insight. This book weaves ancient knowledge into modern life with a clarity and simplicity that belies the profound value it offers.'

– JEREMY SWEENEY, *Former Chair of Trustees*
of the School of Five Element Acupuncture

ON BEING A
FIVE ELEMENT
ACUPUNCTURIST

NORA FRANGLEN

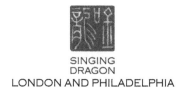

SINGING
DRAGON
LONDON AND PHILADELPHIA

First published in 2015
by Singing Dragon
an imprint of Jessica Kingsley Publishers
73 Collier Street
London N1 9BE, UK
and
400 Market Street, Suite 400
Philadelphia, PA 19106, USA

www.singingdragon.com

Copyright © Nora Franglen 2015

Front cover image source: Shutterstock®

Library of Congress Cataloging in Publication Data
Franglen, Nora.
  On being a five element acupuncturist / Nora Franglen.
     pages cm
  Includes index.
  ISBN 978-1-84819-236-2 (alk. paper)
  1. Franglen, Nora--Blogs. 2. Acupuncturists--Blogs. 3. Acupuncture--
Blogs. 4. Five elements (Chinese
philosophy)--Blogs. I. Title.
  RM184.F58624 2015
  615.8'92--dc23
                                    2014044545

British Library Cataloguing in Publication Data
A CIP catalogue record for this book is available from the British Library

ISBN 978 1 84819 236 2
eISBN 978 0 85701 183 1

Printed and bound in Great Britain

For my family

CONTENTS

Introduction

SMALL WINDOWS
ON THE WORLD

A five element acupuncturist's blog

From my earliest days I have always been fascinated by people, and enjoyed observing human life in all its varied aspects. Perhaps, then, it was not by chance that in my mid-40s, at a turning-point in my life, I chanced upon acupuncture and in particular that branch which, of all others, feeds my interest in human behaviour, that called five element acupuncture.

The world view on which acupuncture is based has guided me to a fresh understanding of the human being, and repositioned me in a new relationship to the natural world. It was as though suddenly the study of the five elements which underlie all Chinese philosophy and thus traditional Chinese medicine helped me view the motivation for human behaviour in completely different terms from the Western medical view with which I had grown up.

The fascination of the new world opening up to me made me look around with fresh eyes, and gave me the desire to start writing, first my books and then my blog, on which this book is based. Blogging has allowed me full rein to express my interest in the complexities of human beings, enabling me to intersperse thoughts about my work with observations on the oddities of human behaviour. No other form of writing encourages such serendipity. Unlike the more rigid structure of a book it has given me the freedom to roam widely through odd byways of thought and up delightful alleyways which sometimes lead nowhere, but offer often amusing insights into the kinds of quirky areas of life which help lighten the all-too serious aspects of my life as a five element acupuncturist.

Writing a blog has proved very rewarding to me. It is each time a little like writing a page of a diary. The pressure of a daily audience for my thoughts out there, some of whom declare themselves to me, others just forming rows of silent listeners surrounding me, stimulates me in my thinking. Certainly the presence of my blog has changed how I approach my writing and spiced it with some urgency, because of the need to add to it at regular intervals.

So here's to further happy blogging.

2010 BLOGS

It's good that I start this section of blogs on the optimistic note introduced by the blog below, and I finish the blogs I have included in this book on a similar note. My fear has always been that the very profound benefits five element acupuncture can bring those it treats may become submerged by the tide of Western medicine-oriented branches of acupuncture which at one stage threatened its survival. No more, I am glad to say. Now, at the time of publishing this book, 2015, this is clearly no longer the case. So this book can in one sense be seen as a paean of praise for what I have dedicated the last 30 years of my life to.

◇◇◇◇◇◇◇◇

5 MARCH 2010

'Remember, Nora, five element acupuncture has been going for 2000 years. It won't die out now'

Isn't it interesting how things come towards us, old or new acquaintances encountered, words written or spoken, as though intended to move us on just at the right moment? Just such a thing happened yesterday, when I read an interview with Arnaud Versluys in the latest edition of *EJOM*, the *European Journal of Oriental Medicine* (Vol 6, No 3, 2009), which has just landed in my letter box. I went to a seminar given by him at the Rothenburg conference a few years ago, and remember listening as other TCM practitioners, not brought up in a five element tradition, showed their fascination with what were, to them, the new ideas in his talk on energy transfers across the five element circle, and thinking to myself, 'but this is what I do every day in my practice'.

Some of what he says in this interview resonates so strongly with my thinking that it has helped reinvigorate my hope for the future of acupuncture.

'...the structure of our medicine is a non-linear, very chaotic structure. It's not even designed to be known completely. That's why I strongly advocate that individual practitioners commit to one style of practice.'

'By virtue of practitioners focusing on one style, they would be really good at what they do and they wouldn't be spread so thin. Because now everybody is spread way too thin.'

But again, on a darker note, 'The future of Chinese medicine is dark, cold and basically one of death. We have a few generations left if we are lucky. I don't see that there is a prosperous, bright future for Chinese medicine.'

His take on the future is understandable, given the acupuncture environment in which he received his training in China, in which a kind of sterile orthodoxy rules, unfortunately like much acupuncture training in the UK. I am not so pessimistic, although I, too, have had many dark moments in my fight for five element acupuncture. My fears have dimmed somewhat over the past year, because I have seen evidence that the kind of teaching I received, and, I hope, passed on, has borne greater fruit than I at one point thought possible.

For I was fortunate, as Arnaud Versluys has been, to learn from a great clinical master, JR Worsley, with more knowledge in his sensitive finger-tips than any textbook could ever teach. And as I have seen the lineage to which he was heir strengthen and develop in the last years in particular, so my fears have lessened.

To encourage me in my hopes, I always hear JR saying to me, 'Remember, Nora, five element acupuncture has been going for 2000 years. It won't die out now.'

◇◇◇◇◇◇◇◇

14 MARCH 2010
Coffee shops I have known

I find that I tend to orientate myself in any town I visit, and above all in the one I live in, London, by the stopping-places for coffee I have found for myself. Somewhere something of my Viennese birthright remains in me, though the Austrian side of my family was forced to leave Vienna when I was very tiny, bringing with it some of the mystique which surrounds that old Viennese institution, the Kaffeehaus. It still evokes for me images of a place where writers and musicians gathered, newspapers were read and society mingled over cups of coffee laced with cream and accompanied by Sachertorte, that special Viennese chocolate cake.

Such places have now become for me places of work, in which I have written all the first drafts of my books. I write in short bursts, by hand, perhaps a page or at the most two at a time, then turn to a book I am always reading, coffee cup in hand to complete my daily ritual. What I look for is a corner where I can tuck myself away, good espresso with a touch of hot milk, and, if possible no music, although silence is increasingly difficult to find. I often only drink one small sip at a time, leaving much of it in the cup, for it is the smell that I savour, the bitter-sweet smell of sweetened coffee, an adrenal rush if ever there is one, giving a boost for my thoughts. I like the anonymity of a public place where nobody knows me, and nobody can contact me. I add steadily to my stock of cafés, exploring new ones, discarding old ones, and have become a great source of knowledge about these staging-posts for my friends.

My accountant has baulked at including the cost of these trips to the café in my accounts, although of all things that support my writing these tiny cups of the cheapest coffee are, in my view, by far the most legitimate expense, far outweighing such mundane things as stationery or travel. But there we are. I will continue to bear the costs without complaining, knowing as I do that the presence of each tiny cup on the table in front of me is as essential to my writing as the computer with which I transcribe the handwritten pages emerging slowly on the table next to them.

It occurs to me that it would be fitting if I dedicated each of my books to the café in which I spent the greatest time writing it, a different one for each book, much as the writer Russell Hoban did for the restaurants in which he wrote his books. To the coffee houses of London I therefore herewith dedicate my books.

◇◇◇◇◇◇◇◇

2 APRIL 2010

A sphere of thought stretched across the world

There are many ways of passing on what we have learnt to those who come after us, and perhaps this is what we should be concentrating upon as we grow older. It is certainly what I feel I need to do, and one of the ways I am doing this is through this blog. Writing a blog is a form of exposure, an opening up of my innermost being to the world at large, and, for me and for everybody else who embarks upon these forms of communication, represents an act requiring some courage. It is the instantaneous nature of it which is both stimulating and frightening.

These thoughts reminded me of the astonishment with which I read Teilhard de Chardin's *Phenomenon of Man*, written more than 50 years ago, and in which, with uncanny prescience in view of what was to come, he predicted the advent of the internet. He foresaw what he called a noosphere, a sphere of thought, growing up around the world like a membrane stretched across it, over which thoughts would transfer themselves instantaneously, much as though the world had grown the synapses of a gigantic brain. He predicted that a word spoken in Japan would register in a few seconds in Alaska. And this is what happens now. I need only press a button, and all the words on my screen will fly across to the most distant computer tucked away on some person's mobile in the jungle or on the steppes of Russia.

How many thoughts, like seeds blown astray on the wind, just dissipate themselves away to land who knows where?

For those who are not familiar with Teilhard de Chardin, he was a Jesuit priest and a palaeontologist, a rare combination, which led to his excommunication by the Catholic church for his views on the origin of Man. He saw the development of this great world brain as an extension of our evolutionary development, and made me understand how crucial to this was the fact that we learned to stand upright on two legs all those millennia ago. As well as releasing our two hands to develop the miraculous dexterity our ten fingers give us, it led directly to the shrinking of the heavy jaw needed to hold a four-legged creature's head upright, and thus provided our brains with the space to expand and continue to expand. I like the thought that the trouble we often have with our wisdom teeth is connected directly to evolutionary changes as our jaws continue to shrink and our brains to grow, a fact my dentist confirmed. Teilhard de Chardin was truly a visionary.

◇◇◇◇◇◇◇◇

10 APRIL 2010
The Placebo Effect

Concise Oxford Dictionary definition: 'Medicine given to humour, rather than cure, the patient' (from the Latin verb 'to please').

How I hate the word placebo and all the baggage of negativity it brings with it! Not only does it patronize the treatment to which it is applied, but, unforgivably, in my view, it also appears to patronize patients by 'humouring' them, as if it does not matter if wool is pulled over their eyes in this way.

Something which is called a placebo treatment is given this name because in some way it is thought that it makes a patient feel better. But is not that the aim of any treatment? It certainly can't be to make them feel worse. If a patient feels better we should applaud this rather than mock it. Hidden somewhere behind the use of the word is the implication that helping people to better health must somehow involve unpleasantness, an attitude which may well be a legacy of our strange Western Calvinistic upbringing, where what is pleasant is seen as wicked. I also see it as evidence of the Western mind-set determined to mock what it doesn't understand. This is nowhere more evident than in comments like these directed at complementary medicine.

Why, then, I ask, are some orthodox treatments, such as sleeping pills or antidepressants, not also labelled as placebo treatments? Surely these, too, could be said to fall under the definition of humouring, rather than curing, the patient!

Since the main impetus for this blog is my thoughts about my acupuncture practice, many of the blogs reflect new insights into my understanding of the five elements (Wood, Fire, Earth, Metal and Water) which form the foundation of my work. The complexities of human behaviour have always fascinated me, and since the elements within each of us are expressions of our individuality, any new manifestation of an element's work in my patients, in famous people or in me is grist to the mill. Hence many of these blogs are dedicated to an ever deeper exploration of the elements' role in the expression of human behaviour.

For more detailed discussion of the five elements, I would direct you to my other books, particularly *Keepers of the Soul*.

◇◇◇◇◇◇◇◇◇

4 MAY 2010
Allow the elements to surprise us

It is only human to long for a time when we are so secure in our knowledge of something that we no longer need to think about it because it has become so self-evident. I think most of us would like this to be true of our understanding of the elements. We would like to be able to place each in a tightly sealed box, labelled Wood or Water, and think no more about it. It would be comforting to think that, locked in these boxes, are all the different signs, sensory and emotional, by which we recognize Wood or Water in people, and that there is nothing out there in the world at large to cast a different light upon what these boxes contain. In this way we would have built up for ourselves fixed templates by which we learn to recognize the elements: such and such a tone of voice represents Wood's voice, such and such an emotion imprints itself upon all Water people.

Unfortunately things are not as simple as that. We cannot capture the essence of an element so easily. It will slip past such clear-cut categorizations, often surprising us by showing us characteristics we might well have thought belonged to another element, almost as though forcing us to re-adjust our thinking. This is why I say being a five element acupuncturist is not for the faint-hearted, because it requires courage to adapt to the challenges of acknowledging that each of us is much too complex to be boxed into the black-and-white categories traditionally ascribed to an element. Rather than being daunted by the difficulties we have in tracing the elements, we should instead be pleased with their capacity constantly to surprise us.

◇◇◇◇◇◇◇◇◇

28 MAY 2010
New thoughts on Aggressive Energy

I have just been asked a question by a student doing a research project on what we call Aggressive Energy in five element acupuncture. I had written something in my *Handbook* about the fact that there are two ways of draining aggressive energy, one through the Associated Effect (*back shu*) points, as five element acupuncturists do, and another by using a dispersal technique on all needling. This was something I had heard in a lecture by Peter Eckman, author of *In the Footsteps of the Yellow Emperor*, many years ago. In other words, five element acupuncture mainly disperses excess energy through its initial Aggressive Energy (AE) drain, whilst other forms of acupuncture disperse energy over a longer period of time by leaving needles in at every treatment.

This set me thinking about this a little more than I had done before (it shows how teaching helps us learn something new each time). I realized that the fundamental difference between the two systems of approach must stem from a deeper fundamental difference than that of simply being a matter of a difference in technique. In five element acupuncture, apart from in the case of specific protocols, such as the AE drain or treating the dragons (what we call possession treatment), dispersing energy (which we call sedation) is much more rarely used than boosting energy (which we call tonification). In the last 15 years of my observing JR Worsley's selection of treatments, I cannot remember a single occasion when he suggested we sedate a patient's guardian element, although sedation is a technique taught all five element students as a matter of course. I have a feeling that as his attention concentrated more and more upon treating the spirit within the body, as I felt it did over my time with him, so he understood more clearly that the element's spirit which bears so much of the weight of the other elements upon it is overburdened rather than gifted with excess energy. Since five element acupuncture addresses the guardian element predominantly at every treatment in an attempt to strengthen it, it is therefore unlikely, seen from a five element perspective, that this element will have any excess energy left to disperse to other elements.

What does happen though, I find, is that an apparently excess pulse on the guardian element will collapse completely after the AE drain and show its true weakness. Apparent initial overexuberance of energy can often mask a level of deep depletion in this way. This may well explain the fact that I have only had to sedate the guardian element in the case of one patient over the past ten years. The remainder of my practice has concentrated on tonifying, on strengthening, this element's energy.

So much that has happened to me in the past three years of this blog has become focused on the invitation for me to teach five element acupuncture in China to Chinese acupuncturists, with all the profound ramifications for five element acupuncture which have stemmed from this, that there will be many mentions of my experiences in China. Below I describe the first step in this exciting journey.

◇◇◇◇◇◇◇◇

1 JUNE 2010

Five element acupuncture comes full circle

Some things come full circle, and it's nice when this is unexpected. One such occasion was a few days ago at a seminar I gave in the Netherlands. It was a fruitful experience for me because I was there to talk to a group of acupuncturists who came together to learn five element skills from a practitioner, Koos van Kooten, who had in turn come to our courses at the School of Five Element Acupuncture (SOFEA). From there he has moved on, developing his own insights and his own approach, and has drawn in his wake an increasing number of Dutch practitioners devoted to deepening their five element skills. All this is very satisfying to me, and provides just the kind of justification for my work at SOFEA that I appreciate.

Amongst his group was a Chinese-trained acupuncturist, Mei Long, who told me that after much exploration she had come across five element acupuncture and recognized it immediately as representing a calling for her. As part of this calling, she had felt driven to get in touch with a well-established contact of hers in the world of Chinese medicine in China, who still has links to its traditional roots and wishes to strengthen them. As a result of her approach he has asked her to run a week's course on five element acupuncture for acupuncturists in Guangxi College of Traditional Chinese Medicine in Nanning, China.

This person turned out to be Liu Lihong, whose name I had come across whilst looking at the work of Arnaud Versluys. Liu Lihong is said to be 'at the forefront of a Chinese renaissance movement that aims at reviving the depth and the core values of classical Chinese medicine'. This is where things come full circle, for JR Worsley said to an acupuncturist friend of mine, Sarah Matheson, some years ago that 'the Chinese will be asking us to bring five element acupuncture back to China', and it appears that they have indeed at last come calling.

◇◇◇◇◇◇◇◇◇

17 JUNE 2010

A little lesson in the difference between the Earth and Fire elements from today's practice

It is in small differences, and with our ability to pick them up, that much of the secret of our capacity to understand the distinctions between the characteristics of the different elements lies. When we realize this, we can use this knowledge to test ourselves and widen our understanding.

I will give an example of this from my practice today. An Earth patient told me of the feeling of mental confusion she often experiences. As she did so, she lifted her hand and pressed it close to her head as if trying to still the thoughts she said churned around inside her. I asked myself whether this gesture could be considered significant as pointing to something particular to Earth. Would I, of the Fire element, ever make a similar movement with my hand? I tried to mimic this movement and realized that I was using a gesture which was totally alien to me. I wondered why this was, and came to the conclusion that, even if my thoughts become confused, which they often do, I clear my mind by talking, as if translating them into a verbal form is what I need to do before I can develop my thinking. By contrast, what my Earth patient apparently cannot do when she is out of balance is put her thoughts into words. Her hand movement was in effect telling me that her thoughts had somehow got stuck inside her head, and the movement could therefore be seen as an attempt to dislodge them.

When I translated this into the kind of treatment that might help her, I came up with the lovely point, XI (St) 8 (Head Tied), located on her head exactly where she had placed her hand, and with a function we could say perfectly fitted what she needed, which was to disentangle the thoughts tied up in her head. Whereas these thoughts of hers had not yet been processed sufficiently to emerge as words, mine, by contrast, never seem to need this kind of help. Rather it is the words I speak themselves which have to act as sieves for my thoughts, a completely different process, which highlights one of the differences between Fire and Earth.

Such distinctions may seem very slight, but they are significant as pointing to one element or another, as everything is that we do. And one of the best things to do is to mimic the words or the movements of another person to see how far the feeling this mimicry evokes in us can lead us to some new discovery about a particular element. Certainly my experience with my Earth patient today has taught me something both about her and about myself, and thus at a subtle level helped me to a deeper understanding of the contrasting thought processes employed by Earth and Fire.

The following blog is really about intimations of mortality which we have increasingly as we grow older. In my case, too, as I mention below, I suffered both a very minor stroke in 2009 and more recently, in July 2013, a much more serious subdural haematoma of the brain, from which, luckily, I have made a remarkable recovery. The latest bout of ill-health temporarily delayed two planned visits to China and other European journeys, but I am now resuming both. Of course both these incidents have changed me. I am aware that time is inevitably pressing more heavily upon me, making me realize that I must achieve as much as I can as quickly as I can whilst I am able to do so.

◇◇◇◇◇◇◇◇

2 JULY 2010
After listening to Tony Judt speaking on the radio

I heard a very moving radio interview with the writer and historian Tony Judt who suffers from such advanced motor neurone disease that he is now completely paralyzed, except for the ability to move his head and to speak. What was so uplifting to hear was the way he approaches his disability and his determination to continue his work, with the added pressure of his impending death to speed him on.

At a much less extreme level I can resonate with what he said, as should everybody, whatever their age, but it is only as I approach my 75th year, and having a few years ago had a very mild stroke to remind me of my mortality, that I have been made so aware that time does indeed press and there is a need for speed in all that I still have to do. It is as though all the thoughts dammed up inside me and jostling for expression are finding a new focus, and are channelling themselves towards expression in written or spoken words, because there is some compulsion to utter them which has stirred within me with increasing urgency over the past few years.

This may have something to do with the closure of the school (the School of Five Element Acupuncture, which I founded in 1995), and the slight hiatus after this as I took breath to recover and realign my life, and now the feeling of taking off in another direction as though I have much work to do before this right hand of mine, still slightly handicapped by the stroke and a daily reminder of time passing, finally refuses to do my bidding and my thoughts falter and fall silent.

When asked about how he viewed his death, Tony Judt said that he did not believe in an after-life, but believed that the point of his life lay in what he left behind him. On the small piece of wood which is the only thing my woodland burial plot (already chosen and paid for!) allows as a gravestone, it would be nice to feel I could write that, in some small measure, I had achieved what I wanted to do and been able to leave something of all that is within me behind.

I have debated at various times whether it is right that I should express what could be regarded as political opinions in this blog, but I see these opinions as more in the nature of my views on social problems of the time, rather than anything do with party politics. What I regard as important for society forms part of who I am, so I think it is right that I use this forum of my blogs to express what I believe are the wrongs in society as well as all that is good about it, particularly insofar as what is good is usually expressed in the actions of individual human beings. I therefore love the quote from Tony Judt's book in the last paragraph of the blog below. I hope that each of the treatments I offer my patients in some small way 'changes the world'.

◇◇◇◇◇◇◇◇◇

17 JULY 2010

'Something is profoundly wrong with the way we live today': Tony Judt

I have just read Tony Judt's latest book, *Ill Fares the Land* (Penguin Books, 2010), a fascinating and challenging book. Judt is a philosopher and social historian about whom I wrote in this blog on 2 July 2010. His book is about what the title of another book, this time by Will Hutton, the political journalist, on very much the same subject, called *The State We're In*. Basically Judt's thesis is that Margaret Thatcher acted like a scythe cutting across all the gains the UK had made in promoting social fairness since the Second World War, and ushered in an era in which self-interest and the pursuit of wealth were lauded above all other aims, with no regard to their effect on the society in which we live. Hence the financial, and of course the resultant social, disasters we now face. He maintains that this trend was further encouraged, devastatingly, by Tony Blair and then Gordon Brown. I myself can still remember how appalled I was when Thatcher abolished essential social services like the well-functioning youth worker network, and encouraged the sale of school playgrounds to developers, thereby consigning generations of schoolchildren to the streets, with nowhere to go and nothing to do, except, inevitably, to add to our current crime figures.

Judt yearns for the return of a time when the good of society as a whole becomes once again the motivating force of society, rather than profit and the achievement of illusory financial targets in all things. He bewails the fact that there are no outstanding characters in government, let alone in parliament, with the vision and drive to halt the creeping advance of self-interest at the cost of the benefits to society as a whole. Just this week, with the announcement of what looks like plans for the wholesale dismantling of the NHS as we know it, we can see confirmation of that, as the parliamentary opposition which should be fighting on the NHS's behalf is intent instead on pussyfooting about who should be its leader, leaving it effectively leaderless and without a clear voice at a time when a strong opposition is needed to take the fight to the government and hold it to account

What frightens me is the terrifying note of glee, rather than appalled regret, in the voices of those announcing drastic cuts to public services. I have heard no expressions of any true concern for those who these cuts are going to damage most, inevitably the poorest and least able to withstand their effects, nor, as Tony Judt points out, any understanding that the unequal society Britain has become, a society with, appallingly, the worst gap between rich and poor of any advanced nation, inevitably endangers the whole of that society, and not just the weakest of its members. If we value what we should now be fighting for, then a reading of Tony Judt's book offers a lucidly argued condemnation of the direction in which Britain (and the USA) are moving, and constitutes a call for action to halt this downward slide.

This is truly a great and important book. And, thankfully, not a very long book. I read it almost at one sitting. Do read it! And if you want to support your local library in its fight to avoid the closures which now menace all public libraries, then order it through your local library, something I always try to do. I regard this as my small, but I hope important, contribution to helping maintain what I regard as essential social services, and my way of trying, through this blog, too, to change things. In Tony Judt's concluding words to his book, 'As citizens of a free society, we have a duty to look critically at our world. But if we think we know what is wrong, we must act upon that knowledge. Philosophers, it was famously observed, have hitherto only interpreted the world in various ways; the point is to change it.'

I have written many blogs about my four visits to China, for which Mei's visit described below was the precursor. Mei's email to me on her return from this her first trip to Nanning gives a very clear idea of how important this return of five element acupuncture to Chinese shores was regarded by Mei's host, Liu Lihong, and how this led directly to my own invitation to teach in Nanning.

◇◇◇◇◇◇◇◇

2 AUGUST 2010
Mei Long on her return from China

I received an email yesterday which warmed my heart. It is from Mei Long, about whom I wrote in my blog of 1 June, *Five element acupuncture comes full circle*. She has just returned to the Netherlands after giving a seminar on five element acupuncture to Chinese acupuncturists. This is her report, which I quote (almost) verbatim, with her permission to include it in this blog.

'Dear Nora,

I was back to Holland yesterday. A very nice flight. My whole trip to China, my staying in Nanning, all the time I spent there with Liu (Liu Lihong), his family, his students, colleagues and friends, everyone, was simply wonderful! Particularly with Liu. We have had quite some deep conversation (he invited me to stay with his family when I was in Nanning), which was really inspiring, touching and warm.

The seminar turned out to be a success. The very first moment when I got there, "the Institute of Classical Chinese Medicine", which was set up five years ago by Liu and his friend Dr Tang, who is now the head of the Guangxi University of TCM, I was taken! There is definitely something special in the air, everything I saw and experienced, everyone there, every greeting I received, every cup of tea I got, in every small thing they did for me, I could feel it. Something which is very traditional has been carefully kept, valued and cherished in that small but wonderful Institute. I feel their respect, gratitude, warmth, above all, so hearty!

I do believe people are inspired and taken by five element acupuncture. Liu's wife (who works mainly with herbs) and daughter (19 years old) listened to the whole seminar, as well as the wife of the head of the university. They all wanted to learn and practise this style of acupuncture in the coming future! They are serious about it. An acupuncture colleague who has good contact with Liu was also invited to the seminar (she read my letter to Liu early this year). She lives in Chengdu and works more with herbs than with needles, because she always feel that "something must be wrong with how people practise acupuncture here". She was so grateful and inspired by the seminar that when she came back to Chengdu, she switched to five element acupuncture immediately! "Finally I find the way," she said to me. And it was like a whole new world opened up to her. She told me quite some stunning stories of her patients. So she experienced right away how deeply this five element acupuncture can touch people.

Liu, Tang and myself are all quite happy with the seminar. "The fact that five element acupuncture is coming back to China is historic," said Liu. They promise that they will do everything they can to offer the opportunity to those who really want to learn it. I told your story with five element acupuncture, how it changed your life and your passion for the elements, your encouragement to me. China thanks you all, JR and you. Liu said to me, when the time is ripe, he wants to invite you to China! You got the warmest greetings from him. He asked me to give his book to you.

I gave your book (*The Handbook of Five Element Practice*) to the Institute, and I said it would be great to have it translated into Chinese. Liu said we need your permission. I agree it would be wonderful to have Liu's book translated into English. I'm a bit afraid my English is not good enough.

After all I feel so privileged and grateful to be able to do all this. I'm just so lucky.

Love,
Mei'

◇◇◇◇◇◇◇◇◇

12 AUGUST 2010
Metal's griefs

We might think that Metal only grieves for a death, but there are many other kinds of losses we can feel. Its grief can indeed stem from the actual loss of a person, but it can also grieve for what can be as acute, or even more acute, than a loss, which is an absence, a person who is not there for them, either physically or emotionally, such as an emotionally distant parent.

It can also mourn all that it will never have and all that was never there. It can grieve for the things it has never done and will now never do, for what it has never known and for what it will now never know, for the losses it will never make up and the joys it will now never experience.

These are some of the losses which Metal, of all the elements, can experience the most profoundly.

◇◇◇◇◇◇◇◇

12 AUGUST 2010
Qualities of the elements

Fire wants to share

Earth wants to involve

Wood wants to tell

Metal wants to observe

Water wants to make sure

◇◇◇◇◇◇◇◇

12 AUGUST 2010
A characteristic of the Earth element

One of my Earth friends often asks me when talking about another person, 'Do I need to worry about them?', said with a kind of weariness in her voice. I see this as a reflection of her own understanding of her role as supporter of others, the mother role, the person worrying about somebody else, but, also, implicit within the weariness behind the words is the feeling that this is a burden. It contains a question as to whether she has perhaps the right to shrug off this burden, as well as the question as to whether instead she ought to find the strength to bear it. And here I am given a role to play, which I see as elucidating further Earth's need to be given as well as to give. For in her question to me is implied the wish, indeed the demand, that I be the one to take some of the burden, in effect to absolve her of the ultimate responsibility of taking on the burden of worry. By asking the question she has placed me rather than herself in the role of taking the responsibility for providing the answer. Hidden within the question, too, is clearly the hope that I will reply, 'No, you need not.'

Earth, then, can often experience others as potential burdens, as here in this example of my friend, with the fear always that they may not feel themselves to be up to the task of carrying the weight of what they are expected to offer others. This explains in part the plaintive note in an Earth's voice, its singing, sighing quality carrying a demanding tone, a 'gimme, gimme' tone, a kind of sucking inwards, as a baby bird sucks in food. This is how I regard one aspect of Earth's need, and if we describe its emotion as 'sympathy', then perhaps in many instances we could add (in brackets) 'for me, please'.

◇◇◇◇◇◇◇◇◇

12 AUGUST 2010
Seeing life through different eyes

It is strange how differently each of us perceives the events we have passed through and the relationships that have accompanied us through these events. It is as though we each see through different eyes, experience things with different feelings and evoke such different responses from those we encounter that it could almost be said that all these happenings are happening to different people. It could indeed be considered surprising that there are sufficient points of similarity in these utterly differing experiences to make communication between one person and another possible at all, let alone productive, so isolated within our own perceptions can each of us appear to be.

This thought came to me after returning from a family reunion to which each member of the family reacted in quite different ways to discussions of a past most of us had experienced together, and reacted differently, too, to the new relationships now being formed through the inclusion of new members of the family. It was indeed difficult to find a common point of agreement in all the differing perceptions whirring around.

This experience taught me again the value of a knowledge of the elements, because I found that I could use it to steady myself in what often felt like the confusing gatherings I was included in during these few days of family get-togethers. If I could pinpoint the reactions of one family member to those of the Metal element, for example, I was better able to understand the reactions of some of the others to this woman's sharpness, and could visualize more clearly why she had responded to her son as she did, why he reacted to her as he did, and why, then, he still bore the scars many years after his mother's death. And I had similar insights in relation to the elements of other family members, including my own element, and these helped reveal why some of the relationships we discussed had been so fraught whilst others had been peaceful. In shedding greater light on myself, I came away much clearer about what I had found difficult in my earlier life, particularly during my childhood, and what I was still finding difficult all those years further on.

◇◇◇◇◇◇◇◇◇

12 SEPTEMBER 2010
Meditation on mastery: JR Worsley and Wang Fengyi

As part of things coming full circle (see my blog of 1 June), I am now in touch with Heiner Fruehauf, who has very kindly sent me a copy of his interesting article, 'All Disease comes from the Heart – The Pivotal Role of the Emotions in Classical Chinese Medicine' (see his website www.ClassicalChineseMedicine.org). In our email correspondence, Heiner mentions Wang Fengyi, master of the lineage he studied under in China. Wang Fengyi practised in Manchuria during the 1930s, when the region was occupied by the Japanese. Heiner says that he 'imported some of this system to Japan'. Heiner describes JR Worsley as 'a Western Wang Fengyi', and wonders whether there could be a connection between what he calls 'these two masters'. After all, JR received some of his training from Japanese masters.

Apart from offering a fascinating insight into the possible transmission of the five element system, his comment also set me thinking about what exactly we mean by the word master, and in particular upon what kind of person I myself bestow this accolade. (Mistress seems never to have been used in this context, as far as I can see, though somebody out there may correct me on this!) I am very clear in my own mind that JR is the only master of acupuncture I have so far encountered, and that I cannot so far attach this designation to any other acupuncturist. No doubt there are other living masters of acupuncture whom I have not met, or acupuncturists I have met who other people would call masters, but each of us must have our own concept of what mastery means. I must therefore draw on my own experience of just one acupuncture master to help me try and fathom what I personally see as the nature of mastery.

I do not regard mastery as being obtained through the acquisition of a particular skill or set of skills or the result of any kind of particular dexterity, nor as arising simply from a level of intelligence applied to a particular discipline. It is certainly not what is attained by gaining a prescribed qualification. It implies something far deeper and more complex than that. Buried within it is always the sense of something which connects this person to the deeper mysteries of life, and thus to the spiritual, and to what may well lie beyond the reach of those who are non-masters or not-yet-masters. When I think of the word, I have a picture before me of a disciple bowing humbly before his/her master. It is therefore associated with a level of reverence accorded by one person to another, implicit in the term 'revered master'. And reverence can never be bestowed lightly; it always has to be earned.

I do not think you can work your way to mastery. You can work towards proficiency, so that you become increasingly competent at what you do, but mastery is not an acquired skill. It is, in my view, something in the nature of a gift, a God-given gift, I would like to add, from whatever God or power or force created the awesome powers which can reside within one human being, a gift which is only vouchsafed a very rare few. And such people touch those they encounter in very special ways, opening doors that without them would remain forever shut.

I was fortunate to be one of the many whom the mastery of JR in the field of acupuncture touched with an especially inspiring touch. And there was no better illustration of this for me than the time when I heard him going through a list of all the points from his *Point Reference Guide*, one of the five element bibles without which, even now, I could not practise. He talked the class through each point on each official, thus the whole mythical 365, and addressed each point as though offering a greeting to them in hushed tones of love. Hearing this I felt I was being allowed a glimpse of a world in which he wandered at will, but which I could only venture into with his help. I understood then that points spoke to him and communicated with him in ways I could myself only dimly perceive, and which bore little relation to the lists of point functions in the many books now vying with each other to offer often dubious insights into point selection.

I certainly do not think that I can aspire, or will ever want to aspire, to the title of master, nor am I sad about this, having a good appreciation of my own limitations as acupuncturist. A good, competent, hardworking acupuncturist I may be, but the magic of mastery will always elude me. It makes it all the more precious that I have encountered mastery once in my life.

◇◇◇◇◇◇◇◇

28 SEPTEMBER 2010
A lovely Leonardo da Vinci quote

I have just read this beautiful description of the power of human vision by Leonardo da Vinci:
    'Who would believe that so small a space could contain the images of all the universe?'

2 OCTOBER 2010

Long-term five element treatment

Many people appear to be puzzled by what they see as the problem of what treatments to give a long-term patient, that is somebody who returns to us for treatment over many years.

I think this worry is quite unnecessary, because it comes from the mistaken feeling that we need constantly to ring the changes in the points we select. Such a feeling is based on uncertainty and a lack of understanding about what we are doing. We can, I hope rightly, assume that with long-term patients we have by this time worked out their guardian element, and therefore which element we direct most of our treatment towards. Why, then, do some of us think that it is not enough merely to continue treating this element in the way we have in the past, and in the way that has, presumably, led to the good results which persuade a patient to keep on wanting to come to us year on year. Why not simply repeat the cycle of treatments in some form or other, not necessarily each time using the same points, which have in the past led to such a successful outcome that the patient thinks it good to return to us for more?

To help the many people who have asked me to solve what to them is a problem, and to me appears the simplest part of treatment, I have gone through the files of patients of mine who have been coming to me for treatment for some considerable time, in the cases I selected, from six to more than 15 years, looking for examples of treatments for all five elements. I have then listed the treatments I have given them over the past three years. People to whom I have given these lists have told me how surprised they are to see how simple my treatments are. If they were to see these patients, I think they would also think how effective these treatments have proved to be.

The elements which have received all these years of treatments, initially as frequently as once or more a week, now as infrequently as a few times a year, are now so attuned to receiving the support offered them by the needle that they need only the slightest nudge to help them back along the path to balance. If, as does of course happen, life deals a patient some heavy blow, then treatment may for a while become more frequent and more intense again, for example if a Husband/Wife imbalance or Aggressive Energy appear, but again the patient's energy will take a surprisingly short time to re-balance itself compared with similar events happening to a patient in the early stages of treatment.

It is indeed always surprising and heartening for me to observe how somebody who returns to me after an absence of a few years may require just one or two treatments to get them back on track, even though the gap since the last treatment has been so long. It is a sign that the elements have long memories, respond very quickly to the familiar feeling of energy re-charging itself in treatment and yearn to regain balance as quickly as they can.

I hope these thoughts will help those who are unnecessarily worried about the whole question of long-term treatment, and confirm my firmly held conviction that, in acupuncture, as well as in many things in life, 'less is more', a term I heard an Indian historian using on the radio this week. So simplicity, and thus the least number of needles for the least number of treatments, is what we must always aim at. It is quite clear to me that those who know what they are doing, in whatever field they are working, and here in the field of acupuncture, always do less than those who don't, and always do it more effectively.

◇◇◇◇◇◇◇◇

11 OCTOBER 2010

How to learn to recognize the elements in the simplest way possible

I am exploring new ways of helping those who have an interest in learning about the elements. This includes not only those who want to learn how to practise five element acupuncture but those who are just interested in learning more about human nature. My own deepest learning about the elements started soon after I qualified, when I was asked to teach some evening classes, and found myself talking to a whole range of people, from plumbers to retired people and young, unemployed mothers. Looking back, I realize that in explaining what the elements represented for me, and trying to find examples of them in famous people the whole class were familiar with, I learnt to see the elements, not simply as a component of acupuncture treatment, but as one way of approaching the complexities of human behaviour. I have always felt that anybody interested in understanding more about human nature in all its amazing variety can benefit from learning about the elements, whether they then wish to extend this knowledge into the field of acupuncture or not.

So how can I best help people wanting to learn about the elements? One way is obviously to let people observe me or other five element practitioners in our practice room, so that we can point out exactly why we think that person is Wood and the other is Metal. But that possibility is only available to acupuncturists or acupuncture students, and then only to very few amongst these, as they have to live near a five element practitioner, or be happy for us to come to their practices wherever these may be. I do this on a regular basis.

For the person wishing to step for the first time inside the circle of the elements, and needing initially to study on their own for whatever reason, the simplest and, for me, still one of the most rewarding, ways of doing this is to sit yourself down in front of your computer screen and use YouTube or similar little five-minute snippets of interviews with people in the news, as a readily available, cheap and highly effective source of study.

This can be considered the first step in what I think can be called a form of distance-learning course on the elements, something which is so badly needed now. There are not enough courses anywhere in the world which concentrate the core of students' studies on the elements. There are unfortunately many courses which offer a kind of add-on five element component, which I believe does more harm than good in consigning five element acupuncture to a subsidiary or even inferior role. In doing this, they do it a great disservice, allowing students to think they have a training in the elements which they do not have.

To counteract this, and to help those who really want to study the elements in the way they deserve to be studied, I am preparing lists of famous people who in my view represent examples of each of the five elements. Obviously, since I have never personally met or treated any of these people, I cannot say for sure that I am always correct in these diagnoses-at-a-distance, but then nobody can absolutely guarantee that they have got it right, until changes brought about by treatment confirm the diagnosis.

Inevitably, I will be starting with Wood, which from many points of view can be considered the starting point of the elements, the bud of life (although Water, the seedbed of life, is perhaps the real starting point). This Wood list will be in my next blog.

Since writing the blog above, with its suggestions for helping people learn about the elements, I have now revised my *Handbook of Five Element Practice* to include a Teach Yourself Manual as an appendix. This provides much more detailed instruction for those unfamiliar with five element acupuncture and unable to find a teacher or a course to which they can turn for help. Those interested should therefore get hold of a copy of my revised *Handbook*, now published by Singing Dragon (www. singingdragon.com), which will help them take their first steps on the journey towards becoming a five element acupuncturist.

It could be considered brave of me to stick my neck out in the way I am doing in the following blog, and try to make a diagnosis of famous people from afar. Since I do not treat any of the people I list, I can have no way of knowing whether I am right or not in my diagnosis, but I feel it is important to help those trying to find their way in the rarefied world of the elements by giving them some pointers to guide them. Being English, most of my examples come from the English-speaking world, but one of the wonders of the web is that people can download images and short films about anybody anywhere else in the world. I therefore hope that people from other countries can use these examples to find compatriots of their own who show the same characteristics as the people I have chosen.

I offer these names with apologies if further thought and further observation of these people's behaviour subsequently make me change my mind! As I often say, 'to err is human', and any changes I make in future will only illustrate further the need for practitioners to be both humble and flexible, and never think that they always get it right.

11 OCTOBER 2010
Famous people I think are Wood

I think the following people are of the Wood element:

Margaret Thatcher

George W. Bush

Boris Becker

Wayne Rooney

Queen Elizabeth II

Princess Anne

John Prescott

Peter Snow

Rafael Nadal

Claire Rayner

Tips to look out for:

Tight tendons, visible on video-clips, particularly around the lips and neck.

Tightly gripped lips, leading to mouth turning downwards. I suggest you try this out yourselves, and you will find that your whole face becomes rigid. It's very tiring to hold this pose for more than a few seconds, unless of course it is natural to you because you are yourself Wood.

Forceful speech (telling others rather than just talking): each word enunciated clearly. The voice does not have to be loud, as implied by the word shouting, but have a push behind it, even if the person is talking quietly.

A feeling of movement, or of suppressed movement, of energy either being unleashed or waiting to be unleashed.

There can, of course, also be what we call a lack of anger, as evidence of an absence or suppression of some of the positive, outgoing qualities of Wood. In that case, the speech may best be described as a kind of whisper, which may have the effect of making the listener angry because they cannot hear it properly. It is worth remembering that each element projects out on to others the emotion it is itself most at ease with. Wood may therefore be happy to create a level of anger or irritation in others which it has been forced to suppress in itself.

No therapist can help others unless they themselves are aware of their own weaknesses and strengths, and can make sure, as far as is possible, that they do not cast their own shadows over those they are trying to help. Knowing your own guardian element, with all its challenges, is an important step for any five element acupuncturist. I have noticed with dismay that some acupuncturists are reluctant to spend the time and effort it takes to track down their own element with certainty, for many reasons, usually to do with wanting to avoid looking too closely at themselves. Only those prepared to admit to their own inadequacies and try to overcome them have the right to help others. Knowing your own element is one step along this way.

◇◇◇◇◇◇◇◇◇

12 OCTOBER 2010

Does it matter if a five element practitioner is not sure of their own element?

We can only be absolutely sure of our element if treatment focused upon it leads to the kind of profound transformation this element will show when its needs are addressed. But practical difficulties have to be faced here. Many people do not have access to a five element acupuncturist for geographical reasons. What are they to do? You can't ask somebody in many of the 90-odd countries that I gather are now reading this blog to make their way to a five element acupuncturist if there is no-one within reach of where they live who practises this kind of acupuncture.

Depending on how determined a person is to learn, they may decide to travel to gain these insights. Others will have to make do with trying to work out for themselves what their own element is, and what the elements of their patients are. It is worth remembering here that even the great master of five element acupuncture, JR Worsley, started with a blank sheet as to his own and others' elements, and only gradually worked his way towards his deep understanding of the presence of the elements in all of us. I would therefore hope that those who have to carry out their five element studies on their own have the courage to explore the world of the elements by themselves, trying to glean as much information from wherever they can. This is one of the reasons which has spurred me on to write this blog. Even though I cannot come to each of these 90 countries to offer in person my insights into the elements, I can at least try to work out ways of helping with some distance learning, as I am doing now.

So to all those many acupuncturists out there who are showing, to me, a surprising amount of interest in reading my blog, I would say, 'Go to it and explore the world of the elements in any way you can. And if you dare to, and are qualified to do this, lift up a needle and work out your own way of practising. Even something as simple as the Aggressive Energy drain can transform a person's life!'

Also, even if you think you don't really what your own element is, at least you have the right to make an inspired guess. And, if you are a qualified acupuncturist, you can still help others. As long as you follow safe needling procedures, you can't hurt anybody. The worst you can do is to leave the patient exactly as they were before you treated them. And remember, also, that treatment directed at any of the elements, even the ones which are not the guardian element, helps all the elements, for, as the Three Musketeers said, or in this case we can say, of the five elements, 'all for one and one for all'.

◇◇◇◇◇◇◇◇

14 OCTOBER 2010
How should we interpret patients' reactions to treatment?

A person commenting on my blog on Aggressive Energy (28 May 2010) asked the interesting question as to whether acupuncture could cause 'a sudden downturn in a patient's underlying condition'. As usual, other people's thoughts set me thinking, and here are some new thoughts of mine.

Any kind of treatment, from conventional medicine to psychotherapy to acupuncture, tries to change something, and, if effective, will change something for the better. But the processes of change in themselves can be disturbing, and often are, as body and soul have to adapt to a new condition, to a state of greater balance, which they are unused to, or have actually never experienced before. A return to balance is not achieved in some seamless transition from imbalance to balance, but usually through fits and starts, some of them challenging. We and our bodies are creatures of habit, and have grown used to the familiarity of imbalance over the years (and the onset of an imbalance can often be measured in years, not days or months). We may therefore find the changes necessary for balance to be restored as surprisingly difficult to deal with. Ultimately, however, they should be rewarding if we stick with it.

In general terms I have found that what somebody describes as a negative reaction to treatment may in the long run turn out to be a difficult first step on the path towards health. As practitioners, we have to have the patience to accept that all lasting change takes time. As patients, we have to have the patience to give our practitioner the time to help us. Most patients we see have been in and out of doctor's surgeries for years before they come to us. Why, then, do we think we must be able to help them in a matter of weeks, as some of us in our over-eagerness do? I have found that patients are not in a hurry if we are not. A slow, steady, tortoise-like approach is what we should be aiming at, rather than one which hustles us into thinking that it only requires a few needles to overturn years of imbalance. This represents a hare-like approach, and we know who ultimately won the race!

◇◇◇◇◇◇◇◇◇

16 OCTOBER 2010
Famous people I think are Fire

I think the following people are of the Fire element.

All these I think are Outer Fire:

> The Dalai Lama
>
> George Clooney
>
> Tom Cruise
>
> Archbishop Desmond Tutu
>
> Lang Lang

I think these two are Inner Fire:

> Tony Blair
>
> Boris Johnson

I have always found the distinction between Inner Fire (SI and Ht) and Outer Fire (TH and HP) difficult, probably because I am too close to Inner since that is the aspect of Fire to which I belong. This distinction is not easy to make, but other people may find it easier than I do! One way I have found to help myself is to see Inner Fire as sorting as it thinks and talks, which gives its speech a kind of hesitancy to it as it searches for the right words. Outer Fire will give itself more time to think, and, when it speaks, will speak in a more articulate way.

Tips to look out for:

Very easy, relaxed eye contact, which tries to set up a warm relationship with us immediately, and hopes that we will respond with a smile.

A movement forwards towards the speaker as they speak.

Laughing or smiling where laughter or smiles do not appear to be appropriate reactions.

A smile which lingers on the face long after the need for the smile has ended. This is most clearly shown in laugh lines on the side of the eyes which remain there even when the laughter has stopped. It should be remembered that Fire enjoys the warmth a smile gives not only to those it is smiling at but also to itself. It enjoys the act of smiling. Other elements smile for different reasons, but not to give themselves joy.

It is also worth remembering that each element projects out on to others the emotion it is itself most at ease with. Fire may therefore find happiness in creating happy feelings in others which it may not itself feel.

All elements can show joy, smile and laugh, but we have to learn to distinguish a Wood expression of joy, an Earth expression of joy, a Metal expression of joy and a Water expression of joy from Fire's expression of joy. Learning to understand the distinctions between an element's expression of its emotion and the expression of that emotion by the other elements is one of the secrets to a five element diagnosis.

One of the joys I have is using my TV set as a teaching aid. I have always enjoyed watching sport, ever since my father took us as young children to watch the 1948 London Olympics. This blog is one example of how much we can learn from observing those competing in sports.

◇◇◇◇◇◇◇◇

18 OCTOBER 2010

To tennis lovers everywhere: enjoy your tennis and learn about the elements as you do

I have had some fun watching a tennis tournament from Shanghai, and persuading myself that this is part of my CPD (continuous professional development – the buzz word at the moment). But watching sport is really one of the most productive and enjoyable ways of learning to distinguish the elements. People competing with one another show their elements in great relief, and since the cameras are always trained on close-ups of their expressions, we can see every twitch of their muscles and every expression of stress.

So what I learnt from watching tennis this week was what I diagnosed, from a distance, as being the elements of the following players:

Water: Roger Federer and Andy Murray

Wood: Rafa Nadal

Fire: Novak Djokovic (possibly Inner Fire, because his Fire is not the easier, more relaxed kind shown by Outer Fire – he seems too prickly for that)

I think seeing the players from the point of view of the elements helps explain why Roger Federer always finds Nadal and Djokovic easier to deal with than he does Andy Murray, who seems to get under his skin (Water trying to outmanoeuvre Water). From Federer's point of view, Water can flow over and round Wood (Nadal), and can extinguish Fire (Djokovic), but how is it to deal with its own kind, in Murray, where the slipperiness and flow which is one of Water's characteristics meet a similar kind of ability to slip past him and win the point? This is possibly why Andy Murray has notched up more wins against him than anybody else, and won again over the weekend. From Nadal's point of view, he can beat Federer if he is strong enough to push Water aside, but what an effort this requires, where the potential aggression of Wood meets the ultimate source of will-power in Water!

Body movements and shape, also reveal a great deal. Nadal has an almost absurdly powerful body, and moves aggressively across the court, whilst Federer's body, and to a lesser extent Murray's, flows more gracefully, with fluid movements, instead of the forceful, muscular blows with the racquet which Nadal uses to power away at his opponents.

So next time there is a tennis tournament on TV, use it to give yourself a good lesson in the elements as you watch.

◇◇◇◇◇◇◇◇

22 OCTOBER 2010
The mystery of pulses

In a comment on my sister blog on five element treatments, I was asked to include pulse pictures with my treatments. I made a conscious decision not to do so for various reasons, some of which I am sure will raise eyebrows (but then a lot of what I write probably raises more eyebrows than I am aware of!). To do so, I must place pulse-taking in a five element context, and here there will inevitably be differences with the purpose and methods of pulse-taking for other systems of acupuncture.

We take pulses for the following main reasons:

At the start of treatment: to assess the overall strength or weakness of a patient's energy, and to gauge the relative balance of the elements and their officials one to another.

During and at the end of treatment: to assess change (but there are some major provisos here which I will discuss).

It is important to be aware from the start exactly what a pulse picture does not tell us.

It does not tell us what the patient's guardian element (CF) is, sadly, some of us may think, for perhaps this would make our work easier. What it can do is indicate that treatment directed at one element has changed the balance of energy, but not whether this element is the guardian element.

We take a pulse reading at the start of treatment, at various points during treatment if we are looking for some change which will demand further treatment, such as an Entry/Exit block, and at the end of treatment. We have a blessedly simple form of pulse notation to do this, compared with the 27 notional pulses of other systems. We assess whether the energy of one element and its officials is in a state of (relative) balance, which we note as a check pulse (a tick), whether it is depleted (a minus pulse) or whether it is in excess (a plus pulse). We assess 12 pulses, two for each of the five elements, plus two further for the two Fire functions of

Heart Protector (Pericardium) and Three Heater. In each case we feel the pulses at two depths, with all the six yang pulses at the superficial level and all the six yin at the deeper level.

It is rare for there to be sufficient discrepancy between the yin and yang pulses of any particular element for us to need to correct this (by taking from the relatively stronger and giving to the relatively weaker using the junction (luo) point), but it does happen. So, for all general purposes, we treat the two officials of an element as one, and usually, but not always, treat both yin and yang aspects of an element at any treatment.

This sets the scene for our pulse-taking. How then do we assess change? The major proviso here is that energy does not necessarily shift quickly after needling. It can change so markedly that our pulse reading picks it up, but it may not if change is slower and less dramatic. It can take hours, if not days, for the elements to show any improvement, and this lapse in time will be reflected in the pulses. To rely on perceiving a pulse change as evidence of good treatment is therefore not necessarily an accurate way of doing things, and to interpret no change in pulses as a sign of inadequate treatment is just as meaningless.

And this is where we need to learn to move away from a reliance on what we think the pulses are telling us to increased reliance on our observation of possible change in the patient. Does the patient look happier, quieter, pinker, less white, talk less, talk more? All these are, I believe, more reliable indicators of positive changes than any changes picked up on the pulses. And since energy continues to change long after the patient has left us, and is always completely different when they come back the next time, there seems little point in spending too much time on writing down a final pulse picture, which only gives what will be a temporary snapshot of energy in process of continuous change.

So my advice to all those struggling to feel, let alone interpret, pulses has always been to avoid over-reliance on something which is so ephemeral and delicate. Instead, use as many other powers of observation to interpret what is going on with a patient's energy. For example, does my patient look as if they are absolutely desperate (Husband/Wife imbalance, perhaps), even if I can't feel the left pulses as weaker than the right? Do they rub their eyes or ears, even if I can't feel sufficient discrepancy between the pulses of SI and Bl to tell me absolutely that there is an Entry/Exit block there? These are the kinds of aids I use to round out my pulse reading.

We should always remember that our fingers may be clumsy instruments for interpreting the incredibly subtle manifestations of body and soul which pulses represent.

I hope this explains why I don't include pulse pictures.

◇◇◇◇◇◇◇◇

23 OCTOBER 2010
Famous people I think are Earth

I think the following people are of the Earth element:

Marilyn Monroe

Princess Diana

Bill Clinton

Oprah Winfrey

Dawn French

David Cameron

Kate Winslet

Joanna Lumley

Tips to look out for:
In my view, the part of the face which reveals Earth most clearly is the mouth.

It is always important to remember where the superficial pathway, the meridian we use for treatment, runs. In the case of the Stomach, it runs down from the eyes to both sides of the mouth, where the important point, XI (St) 4, Earth Granary, lies. It then goes over the clavicle into the stomach itself. XI 4 is a lovely point literally to help Earth draw upon the harvest stored in its granary and take enough energy to swallow both its thoughts and its food better. I have needled this point on an Earth patient who was repeatedly talking about the same things only for him to fall silent as soon as the point started to do its work.

The deep pathways of both Stomach and Spleen connect to the mouth, too, with the Stomach sending a deep shoot off to (or more accurately, coming from) GV (DM) and the Spleen having its own deep connection passing up from its end point at XI (St) 21 to feed the tongue. So we can see from this why the mouth will play a significant role in defining Earth, quite apart from the fact that it is through the mouth that we feed ourselves, and Earth is all to do with feeding, both itself and others.

Since every part of us shouts out our element to those who have the eyes, ears, nose and spirit to perceive, the mouth, too, will have significance for all elements, but, from my observations, all in different ways. With Earth, it appears to express a need. In its most obvious form, I have described this need as being like a baby bird opening its mouth demanding food. People, too, can seem to be demanding food of us, and this can be what we call the appeal which is apparent in Earth, representing its need for us to give it something. When it is exaggerated, the mouth expresses this as a kind of sulky pout, and we can see this quite clearly in all the famous pictures of Princess Diana from her TV interview. It is worth trying to replicate this in yourself, as if you yourself are crying out for somebody to feed you. And the Marilyn Monroe mouth, with its pout, is, for me, another clear Earth mouth.

So if you find that somehow your eyes appear to be drawn to the mouth, this may be (only may be, I repeat) one way of perceiving Earth. A Wood mouth, too, can tell us something. Its lips tend to remain firmly, if not tightly, closed until they open to talk. It is to the eyes, rather than the mouths, of Fire, Metal and Water that we are more drawn, the eyes of Fire because they are trying to draw us into a relationship with them, the eyes of Metal because they look far beyond us into the unknown, even though they are apparently seeing us, and the eyes of Water which will dart around suddenly if they are startled.

Please remember, though, that these are not fixed rules, but only some guides which have helped me with my diagnoses in the past. You probably have quite different observations on which you base your diagnosis of an element.

◇◇◇◇◇◇◇◇

1 NOVEMBER 2010
The concept of the 'elements within'
the guardian element

At a seminar I have just given, one of the students asked me about how much attention she should pay to what we call, in five element shorthand, 'the element within'. This describes the particular colouring or modification given our guardian element by another element or elements. One way of understanding what I think is a very complex concept is to see our guardian element, modified by other elements, the 'elements within', as being in elemental terms the equivalent of a person's genetic make-up. We each have a unique elemental imprint which consists of our principal element coloured by the unique shadings this element is given by other elements.

A Wood person, for example, will, as we know, have green as their dominant colour, shouting as their dominant voice, anger as their dominant emotion and rancid as their dominant smell. But the quality of all these sensory signs which gives this Wood person the unique qualities which distinguish him or her from every other Wood person is given the element by shadings from other elements. Thus one person's Wood characteristics may be modified by Earth, so that their colouring is a yellowish green, the voice a sing-song shouting, their emotion anger laced with sympathy and their smell a sweetish form of rancid. Similarly, another Wood person's Wood characteristics may have a tinge of Fire in them, so that their colouring is a pinkish green, etc. They may also have an added tinge of Wood, so that their Wood characteristics are doubly accentuated, which we call Wood within Wood.

I have always pictured this as a kind of 'wheels within wheels within wheels', since the Earth within the Wood, in the first example, will itself be modified by another element, say Metal, so that the colouring becomes a more whitish, yellowish green, and so on. This is why no one person has exactly the same tone of voice as anybody else, thus making it possible for a unique voice-print to be picked up by a mechanism activating the opening of a door.

What is important in the student's question is, however, how far all this is significant from a clinical point of view. And since I am, above all, a practical acupuncturist, concerned predominantly with what can help me in the practice room, I feel that spending time worrying about the elements within the guardian element may well be time better spent trying to home in on the dominant element itself, since most of us, myself definitely included, find it hard enough to find what I, rather flippantly, call the 'element without'.

Interesting as it is to speculate as to which imprints other elements place upon the guardian element, the important thing is to find this element, a difficult enough task! From a clinical point of view, it has little bearing on the kind of treatment we select, for it is only in very rare cases that we modify treatment in any way to take account of the element within. It may, though, have a bearing on our perception of our patient's needs. In other words, the Wood patient in our first example may be in need of slightly more sympathy, whereas the patient in our second example may be more receptive to a bit of laughter in the practice room.

◇◇◇◇◇◇◇◇

2 NOVEMBER 2010
Famous people I think are Metal

I think the following people are of the Metal element:

Nelson Mandela

Barack Obama

Victoria Beckham

Peter Mandelson

Laurence Olivier

Daniel Day-Lewis

Anthony Hopkins

Tips to look out for:
Metal people have a much greater sense of stillness about
them than other elements. There can be a complete absence
of movement when they lie on the couch, for example, almost
as though they are like those stone effigies of knights lying
in their tombs in cathedrals. This is not a suppression of
movement, as there might be with Water, as it tries to hold
itself back, but a feeling of withdrawal and detachment from
what is going on.

They make very steady and acute eye contact, and it is
to the eyes that we are drawn, rather than to the mouth,
as we are with Earth. Whilst looking directly at us, and
obviously seeing us very keenly, they appear at the same time
to be looking past and through us, as though searching for
something beyond us. It is in their eyes that the sense of grief
underlying this element is revealed.

When trying to work out whether a voice has the weeping
tones of Metal, it is worth trying to close your eyes and just
listen. Somehow when we listen in the ordinary way, watching
the person talking, I find we can overlook the quiet, yin,
falling quality in a Metal voice. Listened to by itself without
any input from our eyes, it becomes surprisingly flat and low,
and draws us downwards. This is exactly the opposite of the
yang, rising tones of Wood in particular, and Fire to some
extent.

When trying to work out whether somebody is Metal,
it is worth watching how the person is making you feel. Are
you finding that you are somehow careful in what you say,
as though choosing your words carefully in case you may be
criticized? Metal judges; that is its role, to weigh the good and
the bad, and discard the bad. It therefore cannot help itself

from judging us, and we can feel this as implied criticism, although it may not be intended as such. It is, of course, above all critical of itself, but will not take lightly anybody criticizing it. You can laugh with Metal, it can laugh at itself (it can have a very acute, sharp sense of humour), but you can never laugh at it without finding that it withdraws completely from you (and in the case of a patient this may be the reason why they decide to stop treatment).

◇◇◇◇◇◇◇◇

8 NOVEMBER 2010
How nice to feel this blog is finding its way to China!

(This blog follows on from my blogs of 1 June and 2 August 2010.)

Two very heartening developments, which help to offset my deep sadness and uneasiness about the future of traditional acupuncture in the UK in view of the closure of the London College of Traditional Acupuncture and the impending closure of the College of Traditional Acupuncture in Warwick, the college where I received my training as an undergraduate.

Mei, who is translating my *Handbook of Five Element Practice* into Chinese, tells me that Liu Lihong had emailed her to say that 'he hopes the translation of your book will be finished and get published soon, which he thinks is the most important thing of all for promoting five element acupuncture in China'. He told her: 'Imagine 10,000 people out there read this book; even if only one of them finds the truth there, it is still good news. With 20,000 readers, we will at least get two people who want to practise it. Then we get a good start already.'

And I have just received the following further communication from Mei: 'I've emailed some of your blog articles and your new blog (my *Five element treatments* blog) to the students of Liu, who find them absolutely valuable. I think your teachings are exactly what they need so dearly. So your tele-education on five element acupuncture is on its way in China.'

The load of keeping a spiritual tradition alive within the core of acupuncture practice has been very heavy for me at times, sometimes, it has felt, overwhelmingly so. These encouraging communications from within the heart of Chinese medicine in China itself help lighten this load. Though it sometimes feels as if a door is closing in our faces here in the West through over-regulation and mistaken attempts to fit acupuncture into an orthodox Western medical framework, it is good to know that another door is opening elsewhere. And where more important than in China!

◇◇◇◇◇◇◇◇◇

8 NOVEMBER 2010
Famous people I think are Water

I think the following people are of the Water element:

David Beckham

Judi Dench

Rowan Atkinson

Gordon Brown

George Osborne

Michael Schumacher

Bob Geldof

Martin Johnson

Cherie Blair

Richard Nixon

Tips to look out for:
Water people tend to make us feel uneasy, even if they themselves look quite calm. They can have a kind of frozen stillness, which can leap into action if they feel threatened, such as when something unexpected happens. Then their eyes are the give-away. Water eyes are always wary, watching everything carefully, and ready to swivel away to look at anything unexpected which might be happening to the side or behind them. They can suddenly look startled, even though the rest of the face can remain surprisingly still.

I see Water's colour as being of two kinds. There can be a very dark shadow over the whole face, in men often accompanied by the typical blue shadow which Richard Nixon showed, particularly when he was under threat politically. You can then think of the whole face as being dark, even though when you look closely it doesn't look so dark. Then there is the other kind of Water colour, when it has a kind of translucence, so that other colours show through it. I like to think that the dark-bluish colour is the Kidney, the more hidden, deep yin, and the translucent, lighter colour is the Bladder, the more outward-facing, yang part of Water.

I have grown increasingly better at detecting a Water smell. It can be very obvious indeed if there is great imbalance, when the smell of stagnant urine can be quite clear. At a more balanced level, I have found that when I am standing at the couch, what comes up to me is a feeling that I am literally near water in some way, as though near a pond or a bathful of water, and it feels as though there is dampness around. This is when the smell just wafts upwards to my nose. This is certainly not an unpleasant smell at all, which the word 'putrid' seems to indicate, but instead just a rather pleasant dampish smell.

I find the sound of the voice makes me feel a little tired if I listen to it for a long time. It has a droning sound, which seems to hammer away at me, but in a more hidden, less direct way than the force in Wood's voice. Listen to Bob Geldof or David Beckham talking (extracts on YouTube are an excellent way of doing this), and this drone, like a bee buzzing away at us, becomes very clear.

But, above all, feel how you feel in the presence of a person, and ask yourself whether you are the person who is feeling a kind of uneasy fear, and, if so, whether this is the fear in the other person, well-hidden, as Water always tries to hide its fear, transferring itself to you. Water is often mis-diagnosed, as it is very adept at hiding itself behind other elements. When I think I can see many different elements in one of my patients, then I have found it is often Water that is the element underlying them all.

As I read through my blogs again, there are some, such as the following one, that I would choose as being the ones that express my deepest thoughts. These would be the ones that I would like to keep if all the others were by some act of computer vandalism wiped from my blog.

◇◇◇◇◇◇◇◇

11 NOVEMBER 2010
A lineage is a line

A lineage is a line which is never complete. It means a line of transmission, and that line starts before a master of that lineage enters the line and continues after that master has died.

I have translated Jacques Lavier's *History, Doctrine and Practice of Chinese Acupuncture* from French into English. As you know from Peter Eckman's book, Lavier was one of the teachers of JR Worsley, Dick van Buren, Mary Austin and others. Much of what is in what is known as JR Worsley's little black book (no longer published) comes directly from the appendix of Jacques Lavier's book, and presumably Lavier in his turn took his information from some of the masters with whom he studied in the Far East. JR is therefore one in an awesomely long lineage going right back to the pre-Christian era, and hoorah for that.

There is no doubt that JR developed his thoughts during a lifetime's practice. I witnessed some of these developments. He undoubtedly dropped much of the more symptomatic acupuncture which fills the black book and to an extent also what is listed at the back of his Meridian and Points book. For example, when discussing possession, I never heard him suggest we select different ID points for patients 'with depression' or 'without depression'. With my first clinical patient as a student at JR's college, I found weak pulses on both Metal and what I call Outer Fire (Three Heater and Heart Protector). The patient was a Fire CF. I was told to tonify both Metal and Fire. I was also taught sedation as well as tonification techniques as a matter of course. In the years of my observation of many hundreds of patients with JR, he never (not once!) suggested that we sedate a patient.

The clearing of AE and removal of all the other blocks, such as Possession, Husband/Wife and Entry/Exit, all reduce the build-up of excess energy between different elements. These must have been improvements to practice which JR developed over time.

A lineage dies out if it is not fertilized by new thoughts in this way. It is the duty of those taught by a master to develop his/her teachings otherwise they become as sterile as some of the discussions and questions flying around now. JR very rarely answered the many sorts of questions that are asked. As I heard him say once, in one of those profound and cryptic utterances with which masters like to puzzle their pupils, but which force us to go away and think, 'If you have to ask that question, you won't understand the answer.'

I don't like all these boxes people forever seem to be trying to enclose five element acupuncture in, nor all the absolutely rigid rules which we were taught as students. Will somebody take me to court because I always put needles into the Heart AEPs (back shu points) from the start (but with extreme care), because I have found Aggressive Energy on Heart and not on Heart Protector? Shock, horror, to those of us, who were taught as I was, only to put needles in the Heart AEPs if there is AE on Heart Protector. I have also found that by putting the needles in the Heart AEPs, AE then emerges afterwards on the Heart Protector needles! That is something new that I have learnt and which I now teach others to do. Have I thereby deviated from the lineage to which JR belonged? I don't think so. I see it as developing that lineage and keeping it alive.

And one way in which I hope I am helping to keep the lineage alive is through my practice and through my writing, in particular of my blog, which I find is fertilizing my thoughts at an unexpectedly deep level. I like to think that I am encouraging others coming after me to go on exploring and through their own practice developing new ways of practising. As JR said, 'If you had all had 40 years of practice as I have, you would be able to do what I am doing.' That may, or may not be true, for mastery is given to only a rare few, but the thought behind his words is that of a true teacher to a pupil. It is to go out there and do better than me.

◇◇◇◇◇◇◇◇

14 NOVEMBER 2010

The uncertainties surrounding diagnosis in five element acupuncture

I have been reminded recently of an important fact about the realities of being a five element acupuncturist. An experienced practitioner of many years' standing told me that what he finds difficult about five element acupuncture is that its practitioners often appear to change their minds as to their patients' guardian elements, starting, say with working on the Metal element, and after some, or even many, treatments moving away on to Earth. He could not, he said, work in a discipline which offered him so little diagnostic certainty, and he was surprised that I did not find this as disturbing as he did. Instead, as I pointed out, I find it exhilarating that my discipline is open to accepting in this way the complexities, and perhaps ultimate unknowability, of a human being. When I asked him exactly what certainties his own practice gave him, we together eventually attributed this to the fact that his practice concentrated almost exclusively upon focusing his diagnosis upon physical criteria, for which he had learnt specific standardized treatments which hardly varied from patient to patient. Where, for example, did the patient experience pain? If in the knee, then he had a fixed protocol of points to deal with this, which came from his knowledge of the meridian pathways affected, and included additional treatments, such as ear acupuncture or cupping, which he had learnt specifically addressed physical problems.

When asked how he would deal with a patient telling him that he was finding it difficult coping with life, he fell silent and then admitted that, apart from offering some generalized sedative treatment to calm the patient, this was an area of his practice that he did not venture into. This was evidence to me of the different emphases different traditions place on specific aspects of a patient's well-being. The central pillar of all five element practice is formed by those areas of what, in Western thought, we would call psychology. The same does not hold true for all other forms of acupuncture. This may also be one of the reasons why five element acupuncture appears to prompt much heated debate as to its validity and arouse a surprising degree of hostility for a branch of acupuncture which is so completely rooted in the deep spiritual traditions of the East upon which all acupuncture is based. You have only to read the classics, such as the *Nei Jing*, to appreciate how strongly bathed in the spirit were the traditions from which all acupuncture emerged. There was never a split between body and soul as there is on the whole in Western medicine, where psychology and physical medical practices lie far apart, and sadly, too, as there appears to be in modern Chinese acupuncture. To a five element acupuncturist, where no such split exists, or should exist, the emphasis upon a diagnosis based predominately upon physical symptoms therefore represents an oddity, only to be explained by an over-reliance on what appears to be physically there, to the detriment of what cannot be seen.

It may well be that a society over-dependent on the physically observable since the rise of science, and thus symbolically prizing the microscope over the touch of the hand or the glance of the eye, has forgotten how far the microscope only reveals, as it were, the physical dimension of things, but can never, unlike the human touch, reach their ephemeral hidden core. It is here that five element acupuncture approaches the realms of psychotherapy, · the treatment of the soul, and where those who find such an approach either perplexing or disturbing may label it, as one practitioner, firmly embedded within the 'acupuncture treats the physical' school, did, as 'too airy-fairy for me'. If airy-fairy means spiritual, well then I would agree that this is a fairly accurate description, but without the overtone of disparagement attached to this remark. It is the 'airy-fairyness' of what I do that fascinates me, because I regard the intangible inner core each human being possesses as dictating the health of the whole structure of body and soul and, in its response to treatment directed at it, creating the conditions which allow the health of the whole edifice to be restored.

But the practitioner who was disturbed by not being able to 'know' with certainty what element a person is highlighted a valid point which deserves to be addressed. If the elements within us are such subtle manifestations that they are difficult to detect even for those with experience, how far does that invalidate the discipline of five element acupuncture as a whole, and, as corollary to this, what particular difficulties does this present to an inexperienced acupuncturist? Far from invalidating it, I believe it strengthens its right to call itself a true discipline, for it acknowledges all those areas which lie at the heart of human life and give them meaning. As to the problems it presents for a newly qualified acupuncturist, the lesson, here, is to remain aware of the uncertainties our practice arouses in all of us, experienced and less experienced alike, and not to deny their existence or belittle the problems they cause. If uncertainty is accepted as being a necessary component of all healing practices, which I believe it must be, since with such practices we are dealing with the complexities of the human being, we can each in our own way learn techniques for dealing with this, and thus lessen our fears.

My next blog will describe a method I have developed to help me cope better with the uncertainties of practice.

◇◇◇◇◇◇◇◇◇

14 NOVEMBER 2010
My calming routine

I have developed a kind of calming routine as soon as I experience the tension of not knowing which element to concentrate upon. If I am unable to home in on any particular dominant sensory or emotional signal coming from one element above all the others, I will experience that all-too familiar feeling of slight panic at not knowing what to do next, which all five element acupuncturists will, if they are honest, often feel. I then move into a routine which I have devised for myself in which I slow down what I am doing, and try to put myself back in the position I was in when I first met the patient. In other words, I try to see the patient with completely fresh eyes once again. To do this I may concentrate on one of the sensory signals, voice, for example, and just engage in some conversation, not primarily to hear what the patient is saying, but how they are saying it. Or I may make a deliberate effort to smell, maybe by moving the blanket away to get closer to the body. I may also take this as an opportunity to look again at my notes. Doing this helps to insert a pause in what I am doing, since I have to page through the file and there has to be silence whilst I am reading. The patient, lying quietly there, is not aware of any hesitation in me, seeing only that I am absorbed in reading my notes and therefore is more likely than not to be pleased that I am taking so much time and care over them rather than, as I might worry, becoming impatient.

In fact the cultivation of periods of silence when nothing is happening except in the practitioner's mind is a good practice to follow. It allows the patient to relax and the practitioner to think unhurriedly. One of the problems we may all have is in believing that we must always be doing something in the practice room, as though action is always a sign that we know what we are doing. If we don't know what to do, because we are not reading the signals coming from the patient clearly enough to work out what treatment we need to do, we must give ourselves time to think, without feeling that our silence will be interpreted as incompetence by the patient.

I have always been quite happy, too, with admitting to a patient whose treatment appears not to be progressing that, as I have learnt to put it, 'there is something here which I don't understand', and asking them whether they are happy to give me the time to work this out. No patient has ever been anything but delighted that I am prepared to give them so much of my time, and all have been happy to agree to coming more frequently for treatment if I think this is necessary, until I have worked out the direction I want treatment to take. For it is unprofessional if, knowing that we are unsure where treatment is going, we then agree not to see the patient for quite a long time, say a month ahead. This only delays the time we will take to get our treatment focused properly, and does nothing but increase the level of our uncertainty, since we have too much time to worry over our patient, with no feedback from seeing them to help us.

We should instead openly discuss our uncertainty to the patient, and ask them to give us the time to work out what we need to do. In such a situation it is essential that we see the patient as frequently as possible, because this gives us the opportunity of looking at them afresh and with these new eyes seeing the elements within them more clearly. Nor should we worry, as some of us do, about our patient's finances here. We should leave it to them to say whether what may be an unexpected return to frequent treatments is making things financially difficult for them and, if so, perhaps we should consider reducing our fees for a short time. In the long run this saves patients both time and ultimately money since the frequency of treatment now will reduce the overall time the patient needs to come for treatment.

∞∞∞∞∞∞

16 NOVEMBER 2010
Think element, not points

When we approach treatment, our mantra should always be: *Think element, not points*. We know that we treat by needling a series of points, but we must think of these points not as individual stitches in a garment, but as shaping the garment as a whole. It has always surprised me how much attention practitioners seem to pay to individual points, whilst placing very much in a subsidiary role the element upon whose meridians these points lie, of which they form only a small part.

I am convinced of the cumulative nature of working upon an element, rather than the need to rely upon the individual action of specific points. In my view it is therefore never just one individual point which does the trick, and turns the tide of treatment as it were. Rather, there is a gradual accumulation of effect, as the selection of different points on that meridian/element adds layer upon layer to the element's effectiveness in redressing a patient's imbalances. There may come a tipping-point as a result of one treatment, where ill-health turns at last to good health, but it is created, not by the points selected for that particular treatment, but as a result of having, with each preceding treatment, through the selection of one point or a series of points after another, placed weight upon weight on the side of the scales of health labelled balance.

The greater the over-emphasis on points to the detriment of the subtleties of the elemental and meridian networks to which they belong, the more practitioners are reluctant to engage with the elements at the deep level such a relationship calls for. This deep level of understanding helps remove the emphasis on individual points, replacing it instead with what I regard as a much simpler scenario. Here the power of each element and of its servants, its two yin and yang officials, remains always to the fore, with correspondingly less emphasis placed on deciding which of its points to select to harness its energy. All points belonging to an element enhance in different ways that element's energy, each becoming one of the many doorways through which this energy can be directed. This is why it is possible for practitioners to choose quite different points on the same meridian and yet lead to a similar level of improvement in the patient.

If the effectiveness of treatment lies in the cumulative effect of selecting points on the same element rather than in selecting a succession of unrelated, individual points, it is then very much a matter for individual practitioners' preferences which points relating to that element are selected at which stage of treatment. These selections are usually based on the protocols used in the particular branch of acupuncture in which they have been trained or by the individual teachers who have passed on their knowledge to them, and they will therefore vary from school to school and from practitioner to practitioner.

◇◇◇◇◇◇◇◇◇

16 NOVEMBER 2010
Cumulative effect of points

It is good to understand the difficulty of assessing exactly what effect one point has rather than that of an accumulation of points added to the effect over time. A point might, in principle, I assume, prove its efficacy not immediately but after some time, as change can occur slowly. Since our patients on the whole continue their treatment with us from week to week, they will have further points needled which may have added to the effect of what we can call that original point, cancelled it or given it a completely different emphasis, so that it is no longer possible to assess exactly which point did what when. Certainly even if it were only the first point that has this future effect, we will never be able to isolate this for all the above reasons, so unless we are simply to needle one point once and await its effect, without adding any further points for a sufficiently long time to give us some certainty of whether it has had an effect or not, we can never know in absolute terms what the effect of that one point on that one patient at that one time is.

Does it matter? Well, yes, it does, but only if we are trying to assess the value of individual points in isolation and to test the accuracy of the information, all generally anecdotal and handed down, by word of mouth or hearsay, or from traditional sources which have grown up around that point and give it a weight and substance that we have no way at all of assessing. I am, however, emphasizing the cumulative importance of treatment rather than that of an individual point. The long-term effects of points used together, either in combination in the same treatment or in sequence as part of a pattern of treatment, will be observable over time and can thus be attributed, one can assume, to the cumulative effect of all the points that have been needled so far. We will never know whether it is indeed only one amongst many that has been effective, or whether it is the whole lot of them combined, or whether it is any combination of some of them, with some remaining ineffective, as another evidence of the dead wood I mentioned. But at least we can gain confirmation or not about the cumulative effect of the points we have so far needled.

◇◇◇◇◇◇◇◇

16 NOVEMBER 2010
Seasonal treatment

The only seasonal treatment I do is treating a patient's guardian element in the season of that element, and with its own element points, for example, XI (St) 36 and XII (Sp) 3 (Earth points within the Earth officials) in late summer for an Earth patient. No other points, including therefore AEPs (back shu points), have any connection with seasonal treatments. You can therefore do the AEPs of any element at any time on patients of that element.

I know some people give seasonal treatment for patients of other elements apart from the element whose season they are in. In other words, for a Fire patient they may give a Metal seasonal treatment, X (LI) 1 and IX (Lu) 8. I do not do that, as I see it as unnecessarily moving away from the patient's own element. An element in balance should be able to deal with any seasonal changes through strengthening treatment on its own points. But the guardian element is always under greater strain than any other element, and will feel this load particularly in its own season. This is why we try to help it by doubling up the support we are offering, in other words by adding more Metal to Metal in autumn, or more Wood to Wood in spring, which is what we are doing when we do seasonal treatments.

All this applies, of course, to horary treatments as well (treating a Water patient with III (Bl) 66 and IV (Ki) 10 in Water time, between 15.00 and 19.00). And to be able to do a seasonal treatment in horary time is said to be the best treatment of all (you are in effect trebling the amount of help you are giving an element). For logistical reasons, this is difficult to do for some elements (Wood and Metal in particular), since patients would have to come to our practices in the night. JR encouraged us to arrange for several patients to come together during these anti-social hours, which, as a good pupil, I started doing, until I realized that a few patients who had loyally turned up between 23.00 and 03.00 in the night for their Wood horary treatments turned out, with more treatment, not to be Wood after all! I have since, for obvious reasons, not least my own health, discontinued this practice.

The following three blogs all deal with my approach to point selection in one form or another. The interest in writing my blog stimulates my thinking in many ways. As I say in my blog on point names, I see my writing as 'putting new flowers into my practice room'. I like to think of my words each as small petals of multi-coloured flowers adding life to my work.

22 NOVEMBER 2010
Point names, and how far they help us in point selection

The individual site we know of as a point has been endowed since the earliest days with a (nearly) unique Chinese name about whose meaning there is much learned debate in those circles which boast a knowledge of ancient Chinese. It might be considered simple to use a point's name as the basis for treatment, without reference either to the meridian on which it lies or to its anatomical position. This represents to me a crude form of point selection, if used as the main basis for selecting what treatment to offer, for it is to take a point out of the context of the body as an interconnecting globe of energy pathways.

Since I have started translating Elisabeth Rochat de la Vallée's work on Chinese point names, I have become increasingly aware of the complex issues surrounding the meaning of point names discussed in the many classical texts she examines. This has helped me recognize that there are wide variations in meanings attributed in these texts to the same point names. They also show many differences not only as to where some points are located, but also on which meridian they are to be placed.

If there is so much debate in the classical texts, it is understandable how much all of this shades over into the even more complex area of the translation of names into other languages. Linguistic purists may complain that the English (or French or German or Japanese) words may eventually bear little or no relation to the original Chinese character upon which they are supposedly based, but such changes are inevitable, given the journey from culture to culture and from language to language that these names have made. This being so, I think, for my part, that a study of the original Chinese characters, fascinating and illuminating though this is, may well best be left to the historian and the linguist, if I, as a practising acupuncturist, am not to be overwhelmed. What I feel is the most important to me clinically is the rationale underlying my point selection, and how far some idea of the meaning of a point's name helps me in this choice.

Every practitioner will have absorbed a number of points into their practice which they feel comfortable to use, and it is likely that this list will contain points with which we have grown familiar because of their use in the tradition we have inherited. The important thing here is that we develop an understanding of our own concept of the meridian network, with an internal logic we can justify to ourselves as we choose individual points. We must place our point selection in the widest context possible, and develop our own rationale for the points we select. Nor must we forget how many layers of learning seep into us from all the many different people we have learned from, who are trained in the discipline which shapes the branch of acupuncture we inherit. All these different pathways of learning, including what personal interpretation we make of a point's name, together go to form a kind of individual acupuncture heritage, and coalesce to form the understanding we have of what points to choose, making point selection always into a very personal journey of adventure.

The important thing here is to be prepared at any stage to widen both our repertoire of points and our perceptions as to when to use a point. I have often found that another practitioner will mention to me a point they use which may be one that I have never thought of using, or one that has somehow dropped off my radar. Adding this point to those I select from then on reinvigorates me, refreshing my practice, much as if I am putting new flowers into my practice room. Our practice needs constant stimulation with new ideas of this kind if it is not to grow stale. This is one of the reasons why I like writing about acupuncture, because thinking about what I want to write makes me examine every aspect of my practice with a fresh eye, as though coming new to it.

What I write below goes to the very heart of my practice, that 'inner quality' which I hope transforms my treatment 'from a mere physical process into something akin to that which is imparted by a caress'.

This is another of the entries which dot this book, denoting thoughts which, if drawn together into a much smaller book, would distil the essence of what I regard lies at the heart of what I do. Such blogs are like leitmotivs interspersed at intervals throughout this book, as important reminders of what I regard as most essential to my practice, feeding the soul of my patients as deeply as possible with what my own soul can offer to help heal them.

◇◇◇◇◇◇◇◇

24 NOVEMBER 2010
A practitioner's intention

Each practitioner in their own way influences the course of treatment not merely by their selection of the treatment itself but by their very presence and the nature of this presence. This is the quality which should make the insertion of a needle into an acupuncture point so much more than that needed to obtain a blood sample from a hypodermic needle. For, enclosed as it were within the physical action of penetrating the skin with the needle there should be some inner quality transmitted by the practitioner's spirit into the heart of the action which transforms this action from a mere physical process into something akin to what is imparted by a caress.

And that is not too emotive a description of what we do, for at a deep level where the practitioner attempts to engage the patient's spirit, he/she must do that with the kind of gentle warmth we impart to those we love. At the heart of all acupuncture treatment at the level of which I am talking lies love, the warmth of one human being for another, allied here to the desire to help another, which is a practitioner's role. Though the needle is solid, unlike a hypodermic needle, in one way it should be regarded as hollow, offering a channel through which the practitioner passes something more elusive and intangible than a physical substance. Within this lie such ephemeral gifts as the practitioner's experience. This will include the confidence he/she will impart born of this experience, which will include an understanding of the transformation the action residing within points can bring about in a patient.

It is therefore vital to understand that the actual insertion of the needle is only a very small part of the process by which the energy to which the point has access is stirred, in much the same way as the manner in which we touch a child can comfort or frighten it. If we are unaware of this, we become mechanical acupuncturists, going through standard rituals, and our needle is then little more than a more delicate hypodermic needle inserted at a physical level to carry out a specific physical action. But, as I argue strongly, what we do must always have within it something of the spirit, and thus the selection of an acupuncture point and its needling must also always be bathed in just such a spirit. So when I select a point I will already have endowed it with something from my spirit which breathes into it my own understanding of why I have chosen it for this particular patient and for this particular treatment, and when I lift the needle what I intend this point to do for my patient flows from me into the needle.

It is difficult to define the elusive nature of the quality we bring with us into the practice room, which is why one person using the same points for the same treatment as another practitioner may have a completely different effect. There is no doubt that the more focused the practitioner is, the more effective treatment becomes. Another acupuncturist once told me that he was surprised that he did not get the same results from treatment as I did, although he was trained in the same discipline and used the same points for the same reasons. This initially puzzled me, until I realized that, at heart, he had doubts about the efficacy of what he was doing, whereas I did not.

It is important that we do not think that this area of our practice, that in which a practitioner can summon to treatment some quality of understanding they have gained from their experience, is only accessible to the experienced practitioner and might make it difficult for a novice practitioner to carry out good treatment. This is far from the case. It is merely that it is important that a practitioner from the earliest days is made aware of this important facet of their practice, and is thus open to harnessing whatever experience they slowly acquire to guide their treatments in the right way. We can focus our intention to achieve whatever we hope to achieve from the first few hesitant steps we take in practice through to those more confident steps experience helps us to take. Merely being aware that a practitioner brings something all their own to the insertion of the needle which can endow that insertion with something much deeper is the first step in this direction.

◇◇◇◇◇◇◇◇

25 NOVEMBER 2010
'Don't get attached to your giving'

Behind many of our fears as practitioners may lie the concern that a patient who is not perhaps getting what he/she wants from treatment, or whose treatment is not progressing as quickly as they had hoped, may decide that they do not want to continue treatment. We must not allow this fear to dictate the course of treatment. We should always let them leave us with as little feeling of disappointment or doubts about our own performance as possible, and learn to move on quickly.

It often happens that we never know why a patient stops coming to see us. Some few tell us why they are stopping, but many others, usually the majority, simply disappear, probably because they are too embarrassed to tell us why they are stopping. And this can happen after many months or even years of being our patients. The hardest to take are those long-standing patients of ours who either decide to move to another practitioner or stop having treatment of any kind without informing us. These we may never hear of again, and, human curiosity being what it is, we would dearly like to know what is going on in their lives, but may never do so, except by chance. As I heard a very wise Tibetan master, Sogyal Rinpoche, saying: 'Don't get attached to your giving,' one of the hardest lessons we have to learn.

Sometimes we hear news of our patient indirectly through somebody else. One such occasion, which I treasure for teaching me a lot about the effect of even a few treatments, occurred recently. A new patient of mine said that he had heard of me through a good friend of his who had had treatment from me, and who had told him that this treatment 'had transformed her life'. I struggled to remember who the patient was, but looking back through my notes realized that she had come to see me for precisely three treatments many years ago, and then stopped coming. Without hearing what her friend told me, I would have qualified her treatment as a failure, as I did at the time. So we never really know what effect our treatments, and perhaps more importantly our presence and approach, can have. And this episode taught me not to underestimate the power of the interaction between the patient and me, nor of the power of those first few treatments in which the elements are addressed so directly and so vigorously for the first time, particularly through the initial cleansing treatment (AE drain) we give. Sometimes for some patients all that is needed is to point the elements in the right direction through these first simple, but pure, treatments, and leave the elements to continue on the path towards restored health through their own efforts as it were. Other patients may need our support for longer.

It is of course obvious that the nature of the relationship we enter into with our patients is crucial to the success of treatment. Of course a patient will have personal preferences which may have nothing to do with a practitioner's competence, and we have to accept that. A patient must feel at ease with their practitioner, as one of the essential prerequisites for successful treatment. If this relationship is for some reason not right, patients will be reluctant to continue treatment, and the treatment itself will rest on very shaky foundations. The kind of uncertainties an uneasy relationship brings with it can lead the elements to hide or distort themselves, as though a screen has been thrown up between us, and the hesitancies which such unease can create in us as practitioners can confuse our perceptions of how to interpret what we see. We may ourselves be anxious and overlook anxiety in our patient, for example, or irritated and interpret through our own angry eyes our patient's emotion as anger.

The lines of communication flowing between the patient and us and between us and the patient need to be as uncluttered as possible, so that the messages passing along these lines are interpreted according to their true meanings rather than being distorted by kinks somewhere along the way.

◇◇◇◇◇◇◇◇◇

29 NOVEMBER 2010
The pleasure of beautiful things

Yesterday I bought a little circular box which I had seen in the window of a local charity shop and fallen in love with. I was told it was carved out of rhinoceros horn, but I don't know whether that is true or whether it is merely imitation plastic. In any case, if it is made of horn, I hope that the rhinoceros from which it came died of natural causes and was not one of the poor animals now hunted by poachers for just such a piece of horn.

The box is about 3 inches in diameter and about 1½ inches high, and has a little hinged lid with a little carved knob on top. Its tiny brass hinges and the brass studs around its base point to its being quite old. I can't see a modern trinket-maker spending the kind of time needed to work these into the side panels. And it is also carefully lined with slightly worn black velvet which could again indicate an object made at a time when craftsmanship was more readily available and cheaper than now. It is a kind of mottled brown in colour, shot through with cream, and the small panels of its base could indeed come from something circular, such as a horn. I will not know what it is really made of, and when it is likely to have been made, until I give it to a friend of mine who haunts the Victoria and Albert Museum and knows all about these kinds of things.

I have put it on a low table on which I gather precious things I take pleasure in looking at. Here it is joined by a tiny green malachite elephant, said to come from the Congo, and a small replica of the Degas dancer, stretching her hands behind her and pointing her toes. I smile whenever I look at my little box. At a penny a smile, it is surely worth the few pounds I paid for it.

What the writer, Rumer Godden, says here is particularly important for people concerned with healing other people. We have to go into each of our patient's rooms with each of our own rooms to help both our patients and ourselves become 'complete persons'.

◇◇◇◇◇◇◇◇

29 NOVEMBER 2010

Each person is 'a house with four rooms'

I have just bought the second volume of the autobiography of the lovely writer, Rumer Godden, who lived most of her life in India. It is called *A House with Four Rooms*. I quote her dedication at the front of the book:

'There is an Indian proverb or axiom that says that everyone is a house with four rooms, a physical, a mental, an emotional and a spiritual. Most of us tend to live in one room most of the time but, unless we go into every room every day, even if only to keep it aired, we are not a complete person.'

4 DECEMBER 2010
Circles of energy

We know that the elements describe a circle creating all things, including the human body, the energies of one element feeding the next and so on in a never-ending cycle. In the body we usually see this as one over-arching circle linking one element to another in the familiar sequence of Wood-Fire-Earth-Metal-Water and back again. We know this sequence as the Sheng (Shen) cycle, the cycle of production. Within this cycle there is a further cycle which has its own sequence, that of mother to grandchild, the Ke (K'o) cycle, in the sequence of Wood-Earth-Water-Fire-Metal and back again.

Here, then, are two circles of energy within us. There is also a further circle, a smaller reflection of this five element circle, which we often forget about and therefore tend to be much less familiar with. This occurs in the order of the grouping of points we call in five element acupuncture command points, which forms one of the most important, if not the most important, group of points. Command points are on the extremities, between the elbows and fingers on the hand, and the knees and toes on the feet. They lie on the meridians of each of the 12 officials, in a specific order, one for the six yin officials and another for the six yang. Most, but not all, command points are what we call element points; this means that they have a specific relationship with one of the five elements. On each meridian there is, therefore, what is called a Wood point, a Fire point, an Earth point, a Metal point and a Water point. In addition to the element points, the command points include what is perhaps the most important point of all, those we call the source points (yuan points). Of all the command points it is the source point which offers the most central reinforcement for other treatment.

If we trace the sequence of the element points, we can see that in both yin and yang officials they follow the order of the elements, but with different starting and end points. If we move up from the extremities, all yin officials have a Wood point as their nail points and progress through the cycle of the elements to finish at a Water point at elbow and knee, whilst all the yang officials start with a Metal point and finish with an Earth point. The actual distribution of the points along the meridians between the element points differs slightly from meridian to meridian, with a few of what are called non-command points lying interspersed at differing intervals between the command points, depending on the meridian involved. This apparently random distribution of the non-command points is yet another proof of the unpredictability of anything to do with acupuncture, each meridian having a unique sequence of command and non-command points, as though deliberately designed to trip up poor students as they try to memorize them. Even now, I sometimes have to refer to my charts to remind myself of a particular order of points.

To see the line of the command points as ending at elbow and knee, with the line continuing along the meridian with non-command points as though we are tracing the meridian from its extremities up the body or from the body down to its extremities, runs counter to our view of the continuous circling of energy from element to element. Instead, it is appropriate to see a kind of connecting link drawing the energy flowing as far as the elbow and knee back round out again to the nail points and on up again following the sequence of the elements, to form a continuous cycle. Thus the Earth and Water points at elbow and knee can be considered as connecting up again with the next points along the cycle, the Metal and Wood points at fingertips and toes. We can therefore envisage all these element points as creating another unbroken circle of energy, a further but smaller circle of energy within the larger, overall circle formed by the meridian network as a whole.

There is something uniquely symbolic about this reflection of the five element circle on our limbs. No other grouping of points elsewhere on the body has such a similarly fundamental relationship to the five element circle in all its mutually supportive power, as one element follows the other in a mimicry of the larger productive five element circle. Even the Associated Effect Points (back shu points), which have a specific relationship to one element each, do not lie along the back in the five element sequence, being linked in a much weaker way with the points of the other elements, since the ones lying above and below them do not follow the five element order. This helps us understand the importance of the command points in connecting our energies to the cycle of the elements. When using a command point of one element we should therefore remember that we are, in effect, drawing to some extent upon energy flowing within a complete cycle of the elements.

◇◇◇◇◇◇◇◇◇

6 DECEMBER 2010
The body as map

I like to think of the body as a kind of map with the meridians as its roads. The individual acupuncture points are the landmarks placed at varying intervals along these roads, some close together, others more widely spaced apart. Some of the areas of the body more crowded with points can be regarded as our body's villages and towns. These are the energetically bustling areas of the lower arms and lower legs, whilst those expanses punctuated only rarely by points, such as parts of the back, upper arm and upper thigh, represent the energetic equivalent of the sparsely inhabited areas of the earth, such as the deserts of Africa or the mountains of the Himalayas. To select points buried within the contours of such a widely varied landscape of the body is then the equivalent of trying to plot a course through the different regions of the globe. It is good to think of treatment and the individual point selections which go to form a treatment schedule in this way, for it is by keeping in mind the landscape of what we can regard as the human globe that we retain that sense of the whole which is essential to good practice.

Perhaps we could go further and think of each element as being one of the five continents on the human globe, with its two yin and yang officials as two countries on this continent. The routes connecting all the continents together are then formed by the meridian network, with its acupuncture points representing staging posts of various importance and size along what are effectively trade routes, the trading of different sources of energy from one area of the energy network to another. This helps us remember that any action anywhere on our body can never be regarded as an isolated action restricted to that one site of the body, but must be seen as having a domino effect, just as a single domino can topple the whole line as it responds to a knock.

I think this metaphor of the body as globe is a true one, for it not only emphasizes the interconnectedness of everything that happens on the surface of the body and deep within, but it is, importantly, also an appropriate representation of the circle of the Dao which encompasses all that is, and of the unbroken circling of the meridian network within us. Somehow the charts of the body with their seductively straight meridian lines make us forget the circular picture which is in truth how we should regard the body. The energies of the five elements do not so much weave us into the straight horizontal and vertical lines of the meridians our charts show, as draw every part of us into a circular movement, much like the 24 hours of day and night draw time into an ever-revolving circle of minutes, hours, days and years. If we can keep this sense of the circling of energy in our mind when working out our treatment protocols, this will prevent us from falling into the error of seeing treatment as forming a straight line, with only one way of getting from *a* to *b*. Rather, it should be seen as a circular action into which different practitioners will draw different treatments at different stages, but all supporting the circle of energy as a whole. Regarding treatment as something cyclical rather than linear supports my conviction that the order of point selections is not as important in the overall success of treatment as the boost to the energy given by a succession of treatments.

It is useful for each of us to develop a map of the body which is personally significant to us, and learn to accept that the selection of points we feel at ease with will always be personal to us, and need not, indeed should not, mimic another practitioner's. We must not be frightened to own what we do in the practice room, each treatment decision we take, each way in which we treat our patients, all must have our personal stamp upon them because they arise from insights we have ourselves gained. This being so, I will be sharing with you in these blogs some of my thoughts about my own personal body map which I have developed over the years and which I hang metaphorically on the wall of my practice room to help me get my bearings.

◇◇◇◇◇◇◇◇

11 DECEMBER 2010
Points as sites of access to the deep within us

We must not think of points as they can appear on our charts, as something stuck on to the body like pins in a pincushion. They must be seen as sites of access to the energy along a meridian, which in turn creates the pathway which eventually passes deep inside us or comes up from deep inside from the organ in question. A point is therefore part of the structure which creates the body (and soul) over which it lies. It provides a point of entry to it and thus allows us, through the needle, to alter the structure of the body (and soul) in some way. Since all is interconnected, we must remember that no point has an intrinsic value all its own, isolated from that of the meridian from which it emerges. The power of a meridian does not therefore lie in its individual points, but in the energy relating to that meridian to which these points form different kinds of access.

Any place on our body, when pressed, stimulated or manipulated in some way, in the case of acupuncture with a needle, will produce some local effect, akin to that of our scratching an itch or rubbing a painful area, but such an effect will remain restricted to that one small site, unless it somehow taps into the larger area to which a meridian has access. Each meridian reaches down into the innermost workings of an organ and from there spreads up and out back to the surface, where we meet it at the acupuncture point we decide to needle. Each time we needle the surface in this way, then, we must remember what lies beneath, and remain aware of how deeply we can influence these depths by this action on the surface, and how the energies lying hidden in the depths can propel themselves to the surface through stimulation by the needle.

11 DECEMBER 2010

Did points come before meridians?

I find it is interesting to speculate whether the concept of meridians came first, and then the points, as it were, popped up along them afterwards, or whether it was the other way around. Were the points there first and somebody (who?) joined them up, like some dot-to-dot picture our children trace? Historically, as I know from my translations of Elisabeth Rochat de la Vallée's work on the points, there is disagreement as to which meridians certain points were allocated to, and uncertainty as to the lines of the meridians, which were not as firmly fixed as they are now. This would appear to indicate that points came before meridians, but there is obviously no clear answer to any of this. Speculation about this is, however, worthwhile because it prevents us from being too rigid in our thinking, and encourages us to look at things from a different angle, always a good idea if our thoughts are not to atrophy.

◇◇◇◇◇◇◇◇◇

14 DECEMBER 2010

Do seasonal influences play their part in Entry/Exit blocks?

When I find an Entry/Exit (E/E) block, as well as clearing it I always think which officials are in trouble and why this might be. Sometimes we simply don't know, but in most cases I can work out why this particular block may have occurred at this time. I tend to think more of the psychological or physical reasons, rather than seasonal reasons, although I have thought of these, particularly if the block relates to the patient's guardian element. For example, one of the most frequent blocks is X/XI (LI/St) (X 20, XI 1). If it is a Metal patient who is blocked in this way, I think of what the patient can't let go of, or if it is an Earth patient, what the patient can't stop thinking about or transport. But I have only thought about a seasonal connection if the patient is in their element's season, i.e., Metal in autumn or Earth in late summer. It might cross my mind that the block has been exacerbated by the season, but I don't tend to think of the season as causing the block. I will not think about the season at all if I find a block in a season not related to that patient's element, i.e., a X/XI (LI/St) block for a Fire patient in autumn (but perhaps I should!).

But, and it's a big but, I am sure that the extra inflow of energy to any particular element from a seasonal influence must affect in some way how those elements manifest in us, since each element will receive the influence of its particular season, just as it receives the influence of its particular time of day. That's, after all, why we do horary and seasonal treatments. I am not sure, though, how obviously the subtle changes in the balance of the elements as they move from season to season can be detected on the pulses, for example, or even how far they will lead to an E/E block. An E/E block is a sign of a great build-up of energy in one meridian which is unable to discharge it to the next along the Wei cycle. As felt on the pulses, it is a strong build-up, and therefore it seems to me unlikely that a simple change from one season to the next will affect this enough on its own (otherwise we would have E/E blocks all round the year as season changes to season).

So in theory it is likely that there may be a subtle influence of the season on the energies of the different elements, but in practice, in my view, it is only likely to add to an E/E block if there is already a block building up. I don't think we have the means of assessing whether this is so or not, so I think this may always remain a theoretical discussion, without practical proof.

I round off this year of 2010 with some cheery words with which to greet the New Year of 2011.

◇◇◇◇◇◇◇◇◇

30 DECEMBER 2010
New Year's greetings to all who read this blog

I always like to take stock as the year ends and we turn towards the future. And I am doing this here for that part of my life which revolves around acupuncture.

There has, unhappily, been much to be saddened by in the acupuncture world in the UK in the past few months, the saddest of all for me being the impending closure of the college where I trained in Warwickshire, and the sudden disappearance, as though overnight, of two other colleges. Happily, though, there is much else to carry forward into the New Year; amongst these things, to my increasing surprise, there is my blog.

Being new to the world of blogging, YouTube, Twitter and such-like before I started, I suppose I am more surprised than others might be at how far into the distant reaches of the world my blog has penetrated. At the latest count it has spread to more than 90 countries, and I still find it exciting when I see that somebody from Ghana, Guadeloupe or Kazakhstan has tapped into their computer and found me. What, I ask myself, has made them interested enough in five element acupuncture to home in on what I write? Not only does this stimulate me in sending out my thoughts, but the interest shown gives me daily confirmation that in writing about the elements I am speaking in a universal language understood by all.

And through this blog I am also seeing that more and more individual seekers after five element knowledge, a rare and growing breed, are prepared to search out teachers who answer their needs, and are finding their way to me and other five element teachers. This is the kind of teaching I love, to people who are prepared to study hard, often on their own and in their own time, to explore the elements and learn how to use this knowledge to help others. I am aware that there are many people out there who have no chance at all of finding a five element acupuncturist, let alone a training college, in their country (or even on their continent!). These are the pioneers of the future, just as JR Worsley and his many teachers before him were the pioneers of old in the UK. I hope they have the courage to explore and innovate, as he did, and I hope, too, that the people who need to will find their way to me and to other five element teachers and will ask us for whatever we can offer.

Finally there is the excitement of seeing five element acupuncture on its journey back to China through the efforts of Mei Long and the translation of my *Handbook*. I will end with repeating what Liu Lihong told her. He thinks that the publication of my book 'will be the most important thing of all for promoting five element acupuncture in China... Imagine 10,000 people out there will read this book, even if only one of them finds the truth there, it is still good news. With 20,000 readers, we will at least get two people who want to practise it."* So I greet in my thoughts all those 20,000 people out there waiting to read my book, and I look forward to welcoming the two who Liu Lihong predicts will practise what is in it.

A Happy New Year to all my readers in all the 50 or more countries around the globe. Amongst the many of those in China reading this there may (who knows?) already be Liu Lihong's two!

---

* And as we now know (in 2015), there are many, many more than the two Liu Lihong predicted!

2011 BLOGS

I have now completed a year of writing my blogs, and am pleased that I have had the tenacity to continue writing throughout the year. There have been times when I felt I could not draw on any new thoughts, as though the well of ideas had started to dry up, only for something to happen which sets me off again in a different direction, and once more, a little to my surprise each time, a new blog emerges on the page.

◇◇◇◇◇◇◇◇

3 JANUARY 2011
A lesson in dealing with a Wood patient

One of my Wood patients told me, rather aggressively, that they found my presence challenging, and, being also an acupuncturist, they attributed this to my being, they thought erroneously, of the Wood element. Although I have learnt over the years never to show that I am taken aback by personal comments from patients, I found that I reacted inside myself with quite a vehement desire to answer back sharply, and had to hold myself back from doing so. Afterwards I found that the episode had disturbed my inner equilibrium, and I tried to work out why this was. By dint of some careful self-examination, I realized that this patient had projected on to me her own dislike of being challenged and had in effect made me angry, often the effect Wood can have when out of balance. I then analyzed my feelings to see what they told me about anger in myself and how far my reaction had been unbalanced, before finally using what I learned from this as a way of understanding not only the Wood element better, but other elements within me, such as Water (my fear of the anger) and Fire (my own element's reaction to stress). An interaction of just a few minutes therefore became through this a valuable lesson about the part of me which reacted to the Wood element, as well as about Wood and other elements in general.

◇◇◇◇◇◇◇◇

7 JANUARY 2011
Daily challenges to our Fire element

We may not ourselves be aware of how far each minute of our life lived amongst other people will be occupied with relationships of one kind or another. I will use the example of the brief duration of a typical day's journey into work to illustrate this. We may be surprised to find how many tiny threads of relationships we knit together on this journey, from the moment we open our front door and turn to wave goodbye to our family, to an encounter with a neighbour, the interactions with a newsvendor and a ticket collector, the avoidance or acknowledgement of eye-contact with all those packed tightly with us in the Underground or on the bus, and finally the arrival at work with the greeting of our colleagues. All these involve numerous small or large skeins of new and old relationships being sorted into their different threads. This covers just a few short hours in a 24-hour period at most, and an infinitesimally small part of all the hours in one year in our life, let alone all the hours of all the years in our life.

In each of these encounters with another person, our Fire element's need to establish a relationship wherever it finds itself with other people will be taxed to the full. Just detailing all this activity is quite tiring, but not nearly as tiring as Fire may feel if, during these few hours between home and office, something occurs which puts excessive strain on this element, such as an argument before leaving home, an unpleasant encounter on the bus or the dread of a meeting with a feared colleague. The constant level of hard work needed to help the Fire element in each one of us in its task of adjusting to all the demands others make upon us places a particular strain upon Fire people, for of all the elements this is the one which most ardently (oh, such a Fire word!) desires to make these relationships work. That is, after all, what it regards as the main purpose of its existence.

What then, are the ways in which we can help Fire in its relationships? To a Fire person the answer appears so simple; it is by allowing Fire people to make us happy, in other words, allowing them in some way to give us something. Fire wants the recipient of its gifts to be happy to receive them, even when we may not ourselves have asked for them. Fire may not consider how appropriate its gifts are, in fact will only do so in states of great balance, for it may be so intent on the gesture of giving that it does not have time to gauge how its recipient is reacting. Nor is it gratitude that Fire is asking for. Instead it seeks the smile and warmth of eye in another person, and, if denied this, will experience this as a slap in the face, a rejection, something which can scar its heart.

◇◇◇◇◇◇◇◇

10 JANUARY 2011
Fears patients may have

If we are honest, we must acknowledge that we all feel some slight apprehension at meeting a person for the first time, particularly when we are about to embark on some form of therapy, where the therapist takes on the role of the person who knows. We may feel we take on a somewhat subservient role, of the person to whom something will be done, about which we at first know very little. In the case of acupuncture, there is the additional fear of the needle itself, instilled within all of us from our earliest days of sitting on our mother's knee and submitting to the pain of vaccinations through a similar instrument. However much we may try to hide or override this fear as adults, it is always to some extent there, however faintly. In some people, the fear of the needle may be so strong that it stops them from entering our practice room in the first place. All these fears, faint or strong, may set up a barrier to our first contacts with our patient which we need to take into account.

As patients, we also have to deal with our natural fear of exposing ourselves to another person, as our practitioner tries to get to know us. The words 'tries to' are here significant, because, either deliberately or involuntarily, we may resist revealing too much of ourselves in the early stages of treatment if we are uneasy about the kind of relationship with our practitioner this will expose us to. We may not actually tell lies, although that, too must not be ruled out, but we may, as the expression goes, be economical with the truth, saying just enough not actually to tell an untruth, but not enough to tell the truth about ourselves. This means that we will inevitably paint only a partial picture of what is going on within us, which can easily be misinterpreted by our practitioner. It takes a surprisingly long time for a patient to feel safe and confident enough in their practitioner's compassion and discretion to open themselves up with honesty. In fact, I believe that each of us will always retain a part of ourselves which we reveal to nobody but ourselves, not even, or perhaps particularly not, to our nearest and dearest, for many different reasons, amongst them the need to retain our own sense of self-respect. As practitioners, we must always allow our patients the right to keep this private area within themselves hidden to the outside world rather than expecting them to open themselves up to us in total honesty, but we must not lose sight of the fact that it may be there.

This is where our perception of the elements guides us towards what is really going on within a patient, for the elements, unlike words, do not lie; they just learn to hide themselves a little to too intrusive an eye. This is also why we should never rely on words spoken to tell us the truth, but use sensory and emotional signatures clearly to spell out this truth in their own particular way. It is easy for our lips to lie in the words they utter, but not in the way they shape themselves as they are uttering this lie, or the way our eyes can reveal something at odds with the tone of our speech.

I was fortunate to be able to observe my own acupuncture master, JR Worsley, at first hand with my patients over quite a number of years, both in my time as a postgraduate student at Leamington, and also after that in my own practice and on his visits to SOFEA, the School of Five Element Acupuncture, over many years. This is when I learnt the importance of simply observing, rather than of asking questions. I would take my observations away to mull over, and gradually extract from them the essence of what he was teaching us to carry over into my own practice.

◇◇◇◇◇◇◇◇

14 JANUARY 2011
An insight into the teaching of JR Worsley

In all my years of observing JR Worsley with patients, it was very rare to hear him explain in any depth why he chose a particular point for a patient, or more frequently a particular series of points. We were certainly discouraged from interrupting treatment with such questions, and we just got on with marking up the points he told us to use. Occasionally I would hear a gem fall from his lips, but often in little asides, as if I was only meant to hear it if I was really attentive. One such occasion was with a patient who was incontinent, when he lightly touched his lower abdomen and muttered, 'We'd better do something down here for you,' suggesting CV (RM) 2 to me.

I came to see that what we sometimes thought of as his obstinacy in not divulging more about his reasons for choosing certain points was instead a very profound form of teaching from master and pupil. As I have said before, I remember him once saying, 'If she has to ask that question, she won't understand the answer.' Now I understand much more clearly that I was being told that it was up to me to work out the answers, and that only when I had worked things out for myself would my real learning begin

◇◇◇◇◇◇◇◇◇

20 JANUARY 2011
Accurate feedback from a Wood patient

It would help us in corroborating some of the principles according to which we work if patients were able to report precise effects when feeding back on the outcome of any particular treatment, but it is rare for patients' assessments of improvement (or otherwise) to be so precise as to enable us to relate this to any particular treatment rather than to a combination of treatments. To encourage us, however, it does, occasionally happen that a patient may say something like, 'whatever you did last time made me feel marvellous (made my backache better, helped me cope better)'.

On rare occasions, feedback can be even more specific. I treasure still, like some beacon in this particular wilderness, the memory of a Wood patient who, when I needled Gall Bladder 40, described immediately in perfect detail the pathway of part of the Gall Bladder meridian. He traced the movement of energy down to the toe and back up along the outer leg, where with great accuracy he showed me the odd lateral dip the Gall Bladder is said to take at mid-calf, and then continued to draw a path up over his knee to his abdomen, finally arriving at his head, where he said, 'I seem to feel something up here at the side of my eye.' I have had other Wood patients describe the line of some movement of energy along a Gall Bladder pathway in this way, but none so precisely as this. It may well be that Wood, the element which structures us, can feel the structure of its own shape reasserting itself as more energy, like sap in a plant, courses through its pathways. I have not had such detailed descriptions of the passage of energy from patients of other elements.

◇◇◇◇◇◇◇◇

24 JANUARY 2011
Showing different sides of ourselves to different people

On the whole, in our relationships with the people we choose as friends we tend to show only one side of ourselves, the one which fits comfortably with the other person. It is likely that we will have discarded early on any too uncomfortable fits, unless we enjoy punishing ourselves or unless, as I as a young girl found I did, I felt it was somehow my fault that I didn't get on with somebody and persisted in maintaining the friendship long after it stopped adding something to my life. Things are much more difficult with family relationships, because on the whole they are there for a lifetime and we therefore have to learn ways of avoiding those areas we find uncomfortable, and we do this more or less successfully.

With patients we enter quite a different level of relationship. We do not choose them as we do our friends. They ask to see us, and we agree to treat them unless there is any professional reason why we should not accept them as patients. We are expected to enter into a patient/practitioner relationship with them whatever our personal likes or dislikes, for our personal preferences should not play a part here. Whether a patient votes the same way as we do or has religious beliefs that we do not have should not be a reason for our not treating them. There is also something reassuring in the fact that, unlike in the case of our family and friends, we do not need to extend our concern for our patients into that part of our life which lies beyond the practice room. It is one of the signs of a maturing approach to our practice that we learn not to let it overshadow the rest of our life, something which often happens in the early days of our practice, when we may become too preoccupied with analysing every tiniest part of our interaction with our patients. I have often quoted the words of Sogyal Rinpoche, 'Don't get attached to your giving,' but I am happy to repeat them here for they have helped me a great deal maintain the necessary professional detachment without which we may allow our own feelings to cloud our perceptions, and in this way fail our patients.

Learning about the elements has certainly helped to make me more tolerant of other people, as my understanding of why they are different from me and why I am different from them has shifted my approach to many of my relationships with others.

One of the prime reasons I gave for running the many evening classes for lay people at various London evening institutes in the past was precisely because I felt that in talking about the elements I was helping in some small way to reduce the level of intolerance which we often show other people whose needs, aspirations and fears often differ from ours. I have always loved the phrase, 'Everybody is odd except thou and me, and even thou art a little strange,' because it states very baldly what I think most of us at heart believe – that others are odd and we are not, just as those others believe that we are odd and they are not. We can all be called odd, if oddness is understood to mean that we are all unique in our own way. Understanding about the elements helps in this understanding.

◇◇◇◇◇◇◇◇◇

25 JANUARY 2011
Why it helps to know about the elements

Knowing something about the elements can help explain our own behaviour, the behaviour of other people and in particular our behaviour in relation to other people. We do not exist in isolation. Everything we do impinges on those around us, as they impinge upon us. The well-worn cliché about raising a finger here on earth and thereby altering the movement of the most distant star is just as valid in the purely human sphere of our relationships to one another. Nothing I do can leave another close to me untouched, just as they in turn cannot fail to influence me. Often these influences may be too subtle for us to notice, but they are nonetheless there. Sometimes, of course, they are so obviously powerful that some encounters knock us off-balance. We may like to think that we live our lives cocooned in a bubble of self-sufficiency, but we all have growing out from us soft antennae, like tendrils, which touch those passing by us, and these touches shift something in us and change our shape in small or large ways.

If we are to smooth the path to better understanding and greater tolerance, we must not forget how different we are from one another, despite all our many similarities, and, I would say, that we are necessarily different, for this creates the amazing variety of human thought and behaviour. It is surprisingly difficult to understand how others view the world. And to those who differ from us we often react with irritation or perhaps even downright dislike, since our inability to understand their way of thinking makes us judge them harshly. We tend to criticize what is unfamiliar to us, and herein lies the root of so many of our prejudices. If, then, our understanding of the elements helps us to see where these differences are coming from, then we are well on the way to engaging in more harmonious interactions with those around us. And, however basic may initially be our understanding of the elements, even the tiniest bit of knowledge will contribute to greater tolerance, a quality sadly much lacking in the world around us, and therefore all the more to be cherished.

I love writing about the good books I read. I have always enjoyed reading, read very fast, often don't remember the actual events in a book I read, or even its author and title, but always remember the feel of the book. Anybody interested in understanding the complexities of human behaviour should read as much as they can, since good writing will always illuminate some of the dark and hidden corners of the human mind, corners we need to be aware of in our role as acupuncturists.

◇◇◇◇◇◇◇◇

30 JANUARY 2011
In praise of libraries

Libraries are some of my favourite places, and now all the more precious to me for being under such dire threat from government cuts. I have always been a stalwart member of my local library, careful to order as many books as I could through it as my contribution towards helping persuade the local council to keep it open. This year, though, I indulged myself and gave myself the luxury of a Christmas present by joining the London Library, a private library in the heart of London with a 150-year-old tradition on its shelves.

The two libraries, my local library and the London Library, are two very different places, and offer two very different but complementary experiences. In my local library I can be sure to find all the recent bestsellers, the detective stories which I love, and all the standard repertoire of books to be found in any Waterstones. They will also order a surprisingly wide variety of books which they do not have in stock, either summoning them from other libraries, or, quite often, buying them for me, something that I still find amazing in these cash-strapped days, all for some tiny contribution in pence from me.

The selection of books in the London Library, on the other hand, reflects its long history. Its dimly lit shelves are laden with tome after tome, conveying an aura of great scholarship for research-minded people, amongst which, unfortunately, I cannot count myself, but I love the smell of old books, whether I open them or not, cherishing the feeling that within them lies hidden so much that creates what we call our culture. Yesterday I found my way to a book of Mozart's letters, then moved on to browse amongst French novels, before settling down to look at their French dictionaries to help me with my translation of Elisabeth Rochat de la Vallée's work.

Long may all libraries flourish, from the smallest in some village hall to their most exalted representative in the British Library. And we should all fight to keep our local libraries open, for when they close a little bit of civilization dies with each book that disappears with them.

◇◇◇◇◇◇◇◇

4 FEBRUARY 2011
Building up our own library of the characteristics of the different elements

Often without our being aware of this, we gradually draw up a list of the characteristics of each element by which we have learnt to recognize them. These are like our own aide-mémoires, our short-cuts, which lead us to an element. It is worth our while to think a little more about this, as we often follow along what to us is a well-trodden route towards an element without being aware we are doing it, and, more importantly, without checking at intervals to see whether our responses have become stereotyped and no longer reflect the great diversity with which the elements manifest themselves. We should always, as it were, at intervals do a stocktake, and throw out any worn-out clichés about an element which have passed their sell-by date.

None of the descriptions by which I attempt to define the elements can be absolutely clear-cut, any more than the distinctions between one element and another can ever be clearly defined. Like the colours of the rainbow, the elements meld into one another at their edges, so that they will share, faintly, some of each other's characteristics. Though faint, these similarities can nonetheless confuse us, some more than others, and explain the difficulties we all have in distinguishing between the characteristics of different elements. My own greatest confusion has always come from the differences between Earth and Fire, and my least from those between Metal and Water, with the similarities I perceive between other pairings falling somewhere between these two. Other people will find it difficult to distinguish between other elements.

Each of us should remain aware of where our own particular difficulties in differentiating between the elements lie, and use them as warning signals along the path to a diagnosis.

◇◇◇◇◇◇◇◇◇

5 FEBRUARY 2011

A very acute comment about the difference between Wood and Metal

I have a friend of mine to thank for the following comment which I think is worth passing on for people to mull over: 'For Wood people, death is far away. For Metal it is very close.'

The blog below has a particular resonance for me, now in 2014 as I prepare this book for publication, since I apparently looked death in the eye during my recent bout of ill-health. What I find difficult to cope with is not so much the fact of the closeness

I was to dying but that I was completely unaware of how near death I was and was only told about this when I was well on the way to recovery. No memory of those crucial days stays with me, as though that week or more has been wiped clean from my mind. It may sound rather odd, but this slightly disappoints and worries me, as though at one of the most serious moments in my life, my family had to deal alone with their own very real fears about me, but without my help. Nonetheless, the event itself has inevitably changed me in some subtle way, not least because it showed me how close are intertwined life and death.

◇◇◇◇◇◇◇◇

14 FEBRUARY 2011
Matters of life and death

Sometimes we come upon a quotation which sets us thinking. This is what happened yesterday, when I started reading a lovely book, another one of those books that have opened up my mind to further thoughts. It is a biography of Michel de Montaigne, the 16th-century French essayist, and the man who coined the word 'essay' ('essai' means 'attempt' in French) which every schoolchild now uses. The book is by Sarah Blakewell and is called *How to Live: A Life of Montaigne in one question and twenty attempts at an answer,* a lovely title in itself.

Apart from stimulating me to plunge back into Montaigne's *Essays*, it brought me this quotation from his writings:

'If you don't know how to die, don't worry. Nature will tell you what to do on the spot, fully and adequately. She will do this job perfectly for you; don't bother your head about it.'

And this stirred another memory for me, taking me back to the first time I read Sogyal Rinpoche's *The Tibetan Book of Living and Dying*, a meditation on where we should place death in our lives. This quotation from the end of the 20th century gives me much the same feeling as Montaigne's words from the 16th century:

'Dying is no problem. It will happen quite successfully. It's how we die.'

What both have in common is an acceptance that the advent of death is a natural event and something we should slot into our lives, rather than as something which is to be viewed as a dislocation, an abrupt, unwelcome ending to be feared. As an acupuncturist I have had to learn to deal with the death of patients of mine, and have had to work out my own approach. It could be thought, as I did at first, that a patient's death is proof of the failure of my skills, but then I came to understand that I did not hold life and death in my hands; that if it is ordained, by whom and for what purpose we will never know, that a person's life has run its course, then it was my task to help make that ending as fruitful and serene as possible, rather than to lament the fact of its ending.

I find both the words of both Montaigne and Sogyal Rinpoche comforting, bringing death and life into a kind of companionship, rather than viewing them as enemies.

◇◇◇◇◇◇◇◇

27 FEBRUARY 2011
Colour, sound, smell and emotion

I have always had a problem with teaching students how to learn to recognize the presence of an element through the four famous sensory indicators of colour, sound, smell and emotion. I know from my own experience that it has taken me many years to perceive some smells, colours or sounds, and then pin on them the label of one of the elements. Even now, after more than 25 years sniffing at my patients, looking closely at them, listening closely to them, I may still not be able to pinpoint exactly what that particular smell, tone of voice or colour is. I have always felt that I am on much surer ground when I look at emotions, and not just those five emotional categories we have divided the elements into, but the whole emotional weight we carry with us which impacts with a jolt upon those we meet.

Of course we can sift this down into the small words of joy or grief with which we label an element, but our emotional make-up is much more all-encompassing than just whether a person looks happy or sad, since it is the overall impression of the whole of our inner emotional life which pours out from us in all that we do. And since we have all reacted to the emotional impact of other people from the day our mother first smiled at us with love (at least we hope it was a smile and not a frown!), this is the elusive quality with which we are, I believe, more familiar than the way we may or may not have reacted to the colour upon our mother's face, the smell of her body or the sound of her voice. Of course these, too, will have affected our responses in some way, particularly perhaps the sound of her voice, but, unless we are blind or deaf, we are unlikely to continue to be as aware in such depth of all the sensory signals as we are by the signals we detect with our emotional antennae.

I don't think I am the only one to have learnt to rely more on emotional feedback than on that from my other senses, because I see the difficulty those new to five element acupuncture have in seeing, smelling or hearing anything which can help them differentiate between the elements. They appear to be able to attune their emotional responses much more quickly as a way into the landscape of an element. This being so, I think it is a bit unfair for students to be expected to give all four sensory indicators equal weight to start with. One consequence of implying that they should be able to do this is that this is likely to make them feel disempowered from the start, and the whole aim of any training must be to empower.

I certainly felt disempowered in those early days as I attempted to see anything which could be called a colour on the areas of the face I was told it apparently showed itself, the side of the temples and round the mouth. This is not where I see colours particularly even now, but instead I have gradually recognized them as imparting an elemental sheen over the whole body. I use my rather red Fire hand as comparison, and by placing it on the patient's body, I can see how another elemental colour will gradually appear in quite startling fashion on my patient's skin, and there before me now lies a bright yellow body or an ashen white body. If, on the other hand, I lay my hand on a Fire patient, the red of my hand softens into a more gentle pink, as the patient's skin and my skin seem to meld together in harmony. (For any practitioners reading this, try this out yourselves. The leg is an unobtrusive place to do this. You will learn a surprising amount about colour from this.)

Obviously there are people who have better vision, smell or hearing than I have. These are fortunate people. I remember that we had somebody in our undergraduate class who picked up smells with remarkable accuracy, but that was an unusual trait. How we envied him as we struggled to smell anything!

So all people out there trying to trace sensory information about their patients, take heart. It will take some years, but gradually the ability to see quite marked differences seeps into us, so that now I can walk in the street and be shocked at how clearly I may see a very green face, or hear a weeping voice talking in the bus. If we try too hard, though, our ability to distinguish these subtle differences appears to fade. It is far better to let the sensory impressions float towards us. And if, like me, you feel you can more easily diagnose which element a person belongs to through the emotions they evoke in you, then this is a perfectly valid way of starting to pin down the difference between elements, as the emotional signals everybody sends out raise an echo deep within us.

I think it is important to add a little light relief to the serious study of the human condition, which is what most of my blogs are about. So I very much enjoy my little humorous excursions such as the one I write about below, and which dot my blog at intervals to help leaven what could become quite heavy to digest.

◇◇◇◇◇◇◇◇◇

7 MARCH 2011

An unexpected skill – predicting bestsellers

I read a lot, and like to read all I can about any new books which are being published. So I scour the weekend arts supplements in the newspapers to see if anything catches my eye.

To my surprise I find that I have developed a good sense of what will constitute a bestseller, well before most other people have even heard of the author, let alone the book or books that will set him/her on their way to fame.

I treasure the fact that I read the first books of the following best-selling authors at a time when nobody else had. All have made fortunes for their authors and their publishers.

Alexander McCall Smith *No. 1 Ladies' Detective Agency*

Stieg Larsson *The Girl with the Dragon Tattoo*

JK Rowling *Harry Potter and the Philosopher's Stone*

Edmund de Waal *The Hare with the Amber Eyes*

I must admit that I gave up on the Larsson books two-thirds of the way through what I considered to be the rather heavy-going second book, though people tell me that the third book is the best, so I may try again.

I got ten pages into the first *Harry Potter*, when I happened to pick it up in the children's section of the library, before sadly putting it down again unread when I realized that it was not going to be the successor to Tolkien's *The Lord of the Rings* that I had hoped for, far from it.

The de Waal is a magical book, beautifully crafted around a family's netsuke collection as it finds its way from West to East and back again. It has very illuminating insights into the cultures and world events its owners experience. Since these cover my own family's background and experiences in pre-war Austria, it added some poignancy to what I already knew.

It seems that I might have a new career ferreting out the next bestseller for some publisher when my acupuncturist's skills dim.

◇◇◇◇◇◇◇◇

11 MARCH 2011
Exploring ways of teaching
five element acupuncture

I seem to be spending a lot of time at the moment trying to work out ways of teaching five element acupuncture now that the colleges who were teaching it as their main form of acupuncture in the UK have unfortunately closed or are in the process of closing. The three years since the closure of my own school to undergraduates have been a time of recovery from all the very hard work involved in running a college, and also a time of taking stock as to what I wanted to do with the rest of my life. Somebody asked me yesterday, surprised at hearing how much I still worked, whether I would consider retiring at some point, and the answer to that is an emphatic 'no'. I can't visualize a life in which I am not continuing to practise and in some way to be involved in acupuncture teaching, and specifically talking about my particular love, the elements, and what they continue to teach me about life.

The field of acupuncture has suddenly started to look like a battlefield in the UK, with corpses of colleges strewn around. I predict more may well be under threat as the tumultuous events which are about to descend upon universities hits them too. Seven universities, I read in the newspapers today, are about to fold for lack of funds. This must surely have a knock-on effect on university-based acupuncture courses. I have always felt that we followed universities too closely, and now it seems they are leading the profession up a blind alley. That being so, I feel I must involve myself, perhaps more than I originally intended to, in supporting five element acupuncture wherever I can.

My blogs are interspersed at regular intervals with descriptions of pointers to one element or another, or to one element rather than another, which I have worked out for myself over the years. This is one more example of this. There are several more in the blogs to follow.

◇◇◇◇◇◇◇◇

12 APRIL 2011
Recognizing the Water element

Another practitioner asked me to look at one of her patients yesterday, and I found it interesting afterwards to think through what had gone on in the practice room which eventually led me on to my diagnosis of Water and away from the other elements.

I met the patient in the reception room for a brief exchange of greetings, and observed a quickness of movement, a rapid shake of the head, and an equally rapid dart into the practice room ahead of me. As she went to lie down, I mulled over whether this had taught me anything. I did not feel that she had looked at me at all, and this made me put both Wood and Metal at the bottom of my pile of elements. Wood, I felt, would have made direct eye contact with me, and Metal would have given me a feeling of somebody sharper, more defined, certainly more likely to observe me, rather than of somebody wanting to escape from my presence. So that left Earth, Water and Fire.

When she was lying on the couch I noticed that she shifted quickly away from me as I sat down next to her, and withdrew her hand as I put mine on hers. By now, I thought, Earth would have snuggled into the couch, and would be holding my hand tightly as though drawing me towards her. There was none of that feeling here. So what about Fire or Water? She smiled warmly, laughed quite a lot, perhaps a little too much, but failed to continue to warm me after the smiling stopped, as I would have felt with Fire.

So now I was left with one element, Water, and at last I could feel things falling into place. I observed my own reactions, and noticed that I was surprisingly unsure of myself, as if I didn't know quite what to ask and what approach to take, a sign of the nervousness Water tends to make us feel, as a projection of its own anxiety. Added to this, I could see signs of fear in the rapid eye movements as she glanced quickly at me and away again. And, finally, I thought that I could smell something wet in the room, which is my own way of experiencing Water's smell. On colour and sound I got no particular feedback to help me.

So with Water we started our treatment. What I suggested was very simple, but as always, profound, because we had first to clear a Husband/Wife imbalance. Then we ended with the source points of Water. She looked different as she left, showing that indefinable difference which is often the only evidence we may have at the end of treatment that a patient's guardian element is revelling in receiving the treatment it needs.

◇◇◇◇◇◇◇

17 APRIL 2011

The onset of summer always disturbs me

People are often surprised to hear how reluctantly I welcome the longer days of spring, which for me herald an even more disturbing season, that of summer. Until I learnt about the elements, and about mine in particular, Fire, I could never understand why this was so. Now I can. I see this as a sign of the pressure building up on my element as the energies of nature change in response to greater warmth, first from the uplift Wood ushers in with spring, and then the full blast of summer's warmer days.

You would have thought, I always say to myself, that I would feel increasingly comfortable as my own Fire energy started to receive its boost of increasing yang energy from nature outside. Why, then, does the reverse appear to be true? I find part of the answer to this lies in the feelings of threat I experience as the world out there starts to throw off its clothes to greet the sun. Everything and everybody then opens itself up more, exposing itself to the gaze. And this is the crucial point, I realize. People are everywhere around me, not hidden away as in winter, and this abundance of people can represent a kind of hidden challenge to a Fire person, because of the abundance of potential relationships it offers, as though its Heart may be overwhelmed as it tries to respond to the demands made upon it.

This may seem fanciful, almost incomprehensible, to anybody who relishes the summer, but then I myself cannot understand why people dread the start of colder days in autumn, which I welcome with a kind of relief. Each season will always represent a challenge of some kind, whether welcome or threatening, to those of that season's element, because of the accumulation of energy it brings with it.

Of course, I realize, too, that my response to summer will always reflect the state of balance in my Fire element. I live in hope, therefore that one day I will float from spring into summer, welcoming it with open arms, as others appear to do. 'Maybe this year,' I say to myself.

25 APRIL 2011
The unknowability of another human being

I think that each of us harbours illusions about our ability to empathize with another human being. To do this entirely would mean stepping out of ourselves, out of that envelope which encloses the unique qualities which define us, and stepping into that of another person. The nearest we can get to this is always to some extent an approximation. Even with somebody with whom we think we are very close, such as a family member, we may think we understand what they are feeling only to be taken aback, as I have been on numerous occasions, by something they say or do which appears to be 'out of character'. It is only so in our eyes because we have given them a character which in some respects is not true to them, but is defined by our own perceptions.

The important thing here is to accept as true that we cannot know another person as we can know ourselves. Since a part of another person is therefore always unknowable, we need to take this into account in our dealings with them as acupuncturists. In other words, we should always respect the unique inner core in another human being to which we can never have true access. The patients themselves do, however, have this access, and will open the door to themselves once they are convinced that we are to be trusted not to abuse our position, or to tread with clumsy feet on such delicate ground. We must therefore allow the patient to lead the way, and it is up to us to follow where they lead.

Little wonder, then, given the extremely delicate and complex nature of our first interactions with our patients, that the chances of our getting it wrong are surprisingly high. It only needs one unwise word uttered at the wrong time for the patient's Heart Protector to slam shut the gates to the Heart, creating difficulties in our future relationship with them. Far better, then, not to be too hurried in our approach, but allow both the patient and ourselves time to orientate ourselves around each other.

◇◇◇◇◇◇◇◇

10 MAY 2011
Political power and the elements

I have always been fascinated by observing the political scene from the point of view of the interaction of the elements in politicians. The UK, now, is offering me interesting insights into the different forms of power-play the elements of its leaders engage in. And of all the elements on show in our politicians, the one which engages me most is the Water element.

It is important to remember here that Water likes to do most of its work in a hidden way, like the powerful surges of the tide which leave the surface of the ocean unruffled. In my view, we have or have had three examples of Water in those in power. First, Gordon Brown, an ex-Prime Minister, who fought a deadly, often concealed battle with Tony Blair over ten years to try and gain the ultimate prize. Then George Osborne, now Chancellor, and somebody, as I heard one political commentator say on TV last night, who always stays behind the scenes and only reluctantly comes out into the daylight. And finally, to complete my trio, Ed Miliband, the leader of the Labour Party, again a hidden man, disappearing in the past behind the obvious charisma of his brother, but stealing power by means of what appeared to be a series of hidden manoeuvres, truly a Cain and Abel story.

All three, Gordon Brown, George Osborne and Ed Miliband, show what are to me unmistakable signs of the Water element, a bluish-black colour, on TV at least, groaning, forceful voices with an inexorable push behind the words, and those fearful eyes which show Water's ever-present fear. All three, too, are proof of the Water element's all-devouring ambition to get to the top, allied with an unfortunate capacity to cause unease in those it encounters. None of these people exhibit the ease Tony Blair (Fire) or David Cameron (Earth) are able to draw on in their interactions with the public. Perhaps it is Water's misfortune, that, though the likeliest of all elements to force its way to the top, it can never for a moment rest easily there, as Blair and Cameron did and can, for 'uneasy sits the crown', and its own unease and fearfulness in the relationships it tries to develop with its political colleagues and the public sow the seeds for what may be its inevitable downfall, as it did so spectacularly with Gordon Brown. We have yet to await George Osborne's public fate, and perhaps David Cameron will shield him better and oppose him less than Tony Blair did Gordon Brown. Ed Miliband, still surprisingly so unknown a quantity, appears to be very awkward in his role, making many people already yearn for the days when his brother David, so very much more charismatic and at ease with himself (Metal?), charmed Hilary Clinton.

And, lest you think that Water's power only shows itself in men, I must add to this trio Cherie Blair, the ever-present, watchful presence behind Tony Blair's throne.

And finally, as I have often said, my diagnosis can only be tentative, as I have never met any of the famous people I write about face to face.

Who ever thought that understanding about the elements was only of benefit to acupuncturists?

◇◇◇◇◇◇◇◇

14 MAY 2011

Don't always think a red face is a sign of the Fire element

One of the most frequent mistakes we have all made is to see a very red face on a patient, and immediately diagnose them as Fire. A flushed face, with an even red spread over the whole of the face is never Fire, I have found, but either Wood or Earth.

Fire's red tends to appear in blotches, interspersed with a much paler colour, particularly around the mouth and eyes. Its red also tends to come and go, as happens when we flush, one minute making the face very red, and then dying away so that the face looks pale and drained of colour. I always see this as the Heart, and particularly its devoted servant, the Heart Protector, pumping away to try and bring a good blood supply to the face, but not having enough energy to keep the blood flow consistent.

Both Wood and Earth can have very red faces when they are out of balance, but their red does not come and go in flushes, but stays there all the time, placing a layer of red over the whole face which almost submerges the elemental colour of green or yellow beneath it. In the case of Wood, I see the red as a result of the weakness of the mother (Wood) causing distress to the child (Fire). In the case of Earth, the reverse is true, even though there may be the same effect of flushing. Here Fire, the mother, is unable to pass on sufficient energy to its child (Earth), causing a build-up of Fire in the mother.

The red of a Wood imbalance comes from its child crying out for help, and the red of an Earth imbalance comes from its mother showing distress. The kind of red which appears will obviously be very different in either case, but may, misleadingly, appear to be the dominant colour. So beware of any snap decision about Fire when you see red!

◇◇◇◇◇◇◇◇

15 MAY 2011
The classical pianist Lang Lang – an excellent example of Fire!

For all the people who read this blog in China (and elsewhere round the world), I am happy to be able to point them to one of their compatriots, the classical pianist, Lang Lang, who is definitely (in my view) of the Fire element. You can see that he is trying to stop himself from smiling even as he plays, and is just waiting to burst into laughter as soon as he has finished.

Have a look at him there or on YouTube, and smile at his enjoyment of his music-making and of life.

◇◇◇◇◇◇◇◇

16 MAY 2011
The 'if onlys' and 'what ifs' of life

I have been giving a lot of thought to how each element experiences regret. We feel regret at doing or not doing something that we wish now that we had done or not done.

Each element has its own special relationship to the past, none more so than Metal, where the past is its special domain. It is here that it gets its most important work done, for it is its task to weigh up and evaluate past actions. The burden of regret will therefore weigh heaviest upon it, for Metal people want to be able to say to themselves, 'I have done this well.' It is not surprising to note how often a Metal person will say, 'if only I had done this…' or 'what if I had done that'.

Other elements will feel the weight of regret less keenly, because for them what is past and gone will represent something different. Wood must plan for a hopeful future, and will have the least time to regret what is past. Fire experiences regret most strongly where it involves hurt it may have done to others, and will try to use this to make the present better. Earth is turned more towards itself, and may not have time to indulge in the luxury of going over the past. Water, the great survivor, may have the least interest of all in thinking of its past in its struggles to stay afloat in the present. For Metal, as we have seen, the past represents the place where it must concentrate its work. The 'if onlys' and 'what ifs' of life will therefore place upon it the deepest cuts.

We can find a helpful pointer to these different approaches if we listen carefully to the tense in which we describe the most important events in our lives. I have found that whether somebody talks most in the present, future or past tense is therefore a simple, but often effective, way of helping me reach a diagnosis, to be added to all the many other little signs by which an element reveals itself. The present tense is about things happening now, the future about things to come and the past about things that have already happened, the tense in which Metal often expresses itself. Wood will be happiest saying, 'I will be doing this', Fire, 'I am doing this', and Metal 'if only I had done this'. Somewhere in between lie Earth and Water.

Our guardian element leaves traces of itself in all that we do and say. I have found different modes of speech to be another simple way of tracking its footprints.

◇◇◇◇◇◇◇◇

22 MAY 2011

Everybody, and not just acupuncturists, should learn about the elements

A former student of mine has just told me that she is no longer practising acupuncture, but writes that what she learnt whilst studying with us 'yet remains a profound education and absolute awakening such that it has imprinted my being for a lifetime. I am deeply grateful to you and those years studying at SOFEA.'

This reinforced what I have been thinking for some time now. A desire to learn about the elements should not be confined to those wanting to use them to study acupuncture or a similar discipline, although this is predominantly how they are studied now. To understand how the elements manifest in each one of us helps us become more aware of our own and others' strengths and weaknesses, and thus develop greater tolerance both of ourselves and others. This goes way beyond a concentration upon the needle and where to place it.

If I were to start my life again (and who knows, perhaps I will in another time and another place, and perhaps, too, on another planet!), I would want to found a school of the five elements, with only a small offshoot dedicated to acupuncture, to which all the world would be invited, young and old, and from any walk of life. It still pleases me that one of my graduates who understands the elements most profoundly was a builder with little education but enormous insight. I still remember his brief essay on the elements in which, in the simplest terms, he captured quite perfectly the essence of each element. Here's to you, Errol, and to our years together studying the elements, from evening class to graduation and beyond.

I would love to be able to offer the elements to many more Errols in another life.

◇◇◇◇◇◇◇◇

23 MAY 2011
The effect we have on others

None of us knows what effect we have on others, for the spheres of influence we spread around ourselves are much more extensive than we think. Many is the time that somebody has said to me, 'I remember what you told me…', when I could not remember saying it, or even, sometimes, the person who came up to tell me that I had said it.

And just as many are the times when I have said, either silently to myself or to the other person, 'I remember what you said,' and how far those words had spread their effects on me and around me down the years. One example of this is particularly vivid to me. Many years ago a friend of mine said, 'I would never let anybody talk to me like that,' and I looked at her and saw that nobody would indeed dare talk to her like that. The signals she was sending out were telling those that approached her to beware. This was when I realized for the first time how a person's aura (I would now say that this is a reflection of their element) envelops them so powerfully that it dictates the actions of those they encounter.

This realization has been a profound lesson for me, for it means that the stronger and healthier a person's elements become, the more they will be able to withstand the onslaughts of life and thus act as protection. This is a particularly valuable lesson for a five element acupuncturist, for it confirms that strengthening the guardian element enables the patient eventually to deal appropriately with stresses which before may have overwhelmed them. When in balance, a person's element will be sending out messages to those we encounter telling them that they can go so far and no further. (This is why I like to call it our guardian element, for it does indeed, in balance, protect us from harm.) The protection it places around us may signal its presence often in very subtle ways, a look in the eyes, a firmness in the mouth, but it is so unmistakable that a person who may be minded to criticize may, as my friend showed me, decide instead to keep quiet. This is the way in which balanced elements show their power, and thus does nature, in balance, protect us.

I like examining my thought processes as I write, and in these blogs I realize that I spend quite a lot of time examining the way my mind works and trying to understand through words the reasons why I do what I do. To that extent, these blogs form a kind of diary of my life, containing elements of an autobiography. My work is concerned above all with trying to understand the intricacies of human behaviour, so I use everybody I meet, including obviously myself, too, as food for my thoughts. The blog below is another example of this.

◇◇◇◇◇◇◇◇

10 JUNE 2011

All the little relationships the Small Intestine is asked to enter into

A conference like the one I went to at Rothenburg in Germany last week, with its 1000 participants, makes special demands upon my Small Intestine. The little medieval town is overrun with acupuncturists, making it extremely likely that the person you pass in the street will be a fellow acupuncturist. This presents a particular challenge for anybody who is Inner Fire, like me, for every contact with another person, however fleeting, offers the potential for a tiny relationship to be formed. Each person I passed in the Rothenburg streets therefore placed a slight strain on my Small Intestine as it asked itself how wide it wanted to open the doors to my Heart, or whether it was wiser simply to look away and not engage.

These constant challenges to my Small Intestine meant that it could never really relax, for if it does so it would feel that it is abdicating its responsibility to protect the Heart. Luckily, the meetings with good friends of mine who were also there helped to lighten the load. When I was with them, all was well, my Heart beamed with joy and my Small Intestine could at last relax. But never entirely, however, for it is such a necessarily restless aspect of Fire, and always has to be on the go, sifting and sorting, sifting and sorting.

In an idle moment I sometimes wish I were another element! And if I had a choice as to which one, I think it would have to be Metal, so quiet and self-contained, so able to cut itself off from people without a second thought. It would have no such problems as I have in deciding who to smile at and who to ignore. But then I know that it too, will of course have its own different, but less people-centred stresses.

◇◇◇◇◇◇◇◇

12 JUNE 2011
A lesson in humility

Without our being aware of it, we tend to overlook the shadows our own elements cast over the patients we are treating, and which therefore inevitably to some extent distort the signals our patients' elements are sending us. We all have one (or more) weak spots in recognizing specific elements, and if we are to be good practitioners we must learn to accept this and take this into account in any diagnosis we make. Mine is definitely distinguishing between Fire and Earth, something I find I have in common with many other practitioners. I see that this comes from the fact that both elements, in their differing ways, need people, and therefore respond to people with some eagerness.

In my case, I have come to see that one of the reasons for this may lie in the interaction between my own Fire element and Earth people and other Fire people, and the way in which my own Fire responds when confronting the needs of these two elements. My Fire need is to relate closely to each of my patients, and I will be tempted to interpret the warmth with which both Fire and Earth will respond to my warmth as though filtered through what I call my pink Fire spectacles. But Earth's and Fire's responses differ, as we know. Earth responds more because it is glad to be offered understanding, Fire more because it is happy to bestow warmth upon the practitioner. Both interactions will make my own Fire element happy, but for different reasons. With Earth I am pleased to see that my offerings are being so warmly accepted (we could say, taken in and swallowed), and I will bask in the warmth my Fire patients offer me.

The direction of movement is quite different in the two cases. Earth's is to move back and take in, while Fire's is to move forward and give.

I have been thinking a lot about this ever since a fellow practitioner said to me recently, 'You know that famous film actress with the large smile? I see her as so typically Earth, with that mouth which you, Nora, have often called an Earth mouth, open like a baby bird crying out for food.' She was talking about Julia Roberts. I was taken aback because Julia Roberts is somebody I rather blithely originally included in my list of what I considered to be Fire people. Was it possible that my fellow practitioner was right, and was that, perhaps, the reason why Julia Roberts doesn't actually make me feel warm inside, despite the great smile? So off I went to look at her on YouTube, and indeed, when I looked more closely and more carefully, what I saw was somebody who demanded something of me, rather than somebody who gave me something.

This reinforces one of my mantras. Never allow yourself to be lulled into thinking you are absolutely certain about a person's guardian element, but always keep open the possibility that you may be misinterpreting the signals coming from their elements. And always, always, remain humble and ready to learn. The uniqueness of each person is not easily encapsulated within the all-encompassing meanings contained in one of five words, Wood, Fire…

◇◇◇◇◇◇◇◇

16 JUNE 2011
Meetings with remarkable people

I am fortunate to have had that part of my life, the part into which five element acupuncture burst like some spray of stardust, its second half, illuminated (not too strong a word) by two remarkable masters, both of whom, in their differing ways, moved my life onwards in a different direction, but to me, looking back now, somehow in a pre-ordained way.

The first was JR Worsley, the second now is Liu Lihong. The first led me deep into a world of the spirit which has informed my acupuncture practice ever since. The second has only just appeared over my horizon, but is just beckoning to me from that vast region of the physical world which is China, and from that vast region of the spiritual world which is Chinese thought embedded deep in its past, the thoughts of the Nei Jing, of Lao Tse and of all the long and ancient lineage of practitioners of traditional Chinese medicine.

I started my acupuncture studies because I was curious to understand the profound reactions awoken in me by my own treatment. I only encountered JR Worsley late on in my studies, but my further studies with him, his visits to my practice and my many visits with my patients to consultation days with him deepened my understanding of his profound contribution to moving acupuncture forward into the modern world and widening it to encompass the psychological insights this modern world has provided. He represents the first stage of my encounter with acupuncture.

The second stage starts after I closed my acupuncture college a few years ago, and this was followed by a gap in time, before the next part of my acupuncture life began about a year ago. It was then that I met Mei Long, a young Chinese acupuncturist practising in Holland, and my acupuncture path moved forwards in a different direction, this time towards China (see my blogs of 1 June, 2 August and 8 November 2010). Mei has now completed her translation of my *Handbook of Five Element Practice* into Chinese, and it is now in proof form (it looks beautiful), awaiting an introduction to be written by Liu Lihong.

And here we come to my second important encounter, that with Liu Lihong, which took place at the Rothenburg Conference a few weeks ago. Having written a seminal book, *Reflections on Traditional Chinese Medicine*, which Mei tells me is a bestseller in China, he is determined to bring back to traditional Chinese medicine the spirit which has drained from it, and sees five element acupuncture as representing that spirit in the field of acupuncture (he is a traditional herbalist). He is encouraging me to come to China once my book is published over there, which should be in the next few months. So as one door closed upon my life as a teacher in the UK, the next, beckoning me to continue my teaching in China, now opens for me. My acupuncture life has indeed been fortunate to have been blessed by two such important encounters with remarkable men.

Finally, lest anybody should think that it is only men who have taught me the great lessons of life, these encounters were preceded by one which brought to an end the first half of my life, for this part of my life was illuminated by the insights of a very great woman, Anna Freud, Freud's daughter. She died just before I encountered acupuncture, and she would have been delighted to know the direction my life took not long after her death, for she was always encouraging me 'to do something big'. I think I now dare say, a little hesitantly and I hope with due humility, that I have now done what she would have liked me to do. I am sure that without her encouragement I would never have dared do what I have done or write what I have written, including this present blog! Nor would I have been ready to accept the challenges my life has offered, and might instead have been tempted to turn my back upon them as I would have done in earlier days.

I give thanks for having been granted the rare grace of encountering three such remarkable people, each of whom in some way changed or is changing the direction of my life.

◇◇◇◇◇◇◇◇◇

25 JUNE 2011
'Protecting oneself from the eternities'

I have spent the last days re-reading one of my favourite books, *The Enchanted April* by Elizabeth von Arnim. If you haven't read it, and want to emerge from the last page smiling and at peace, then do. It is a beautiful, heart-warming book. (And the film they made of it, surprisingly, recreates this warmth and beauty wonderfully.)

And, as usually happens when one reads, up popped some words which echo so much that I feel expresses my wonder at the depths and awesomeness of human life.

'She pulled her wrap closer round her with a gesture of defence, of keeping out and off. She didn't want to grow sentimental. Difficult not to, here; the marvellous night stole in through all one's chinks, and brought in with it, whether one wanted them or not, enormous feelings – feelings one couldn't manage, great things about death and time and waste; glorious and devastating things, magnificent and bleak, at once rapture and terror and immense, heart-cleaving longing. She felt small and dreadfully alone. She felt uncovered and defenceless. Instinctively she pulled her wrap closer. With this thing of chiffon she tried to protect herself from the eternities.'

Perhaps we can never truly protect ourselves from the eternities, nor should we. We should be awed by them, often frightened by them, but always, always acknowledge their presence.

◇◇◇◇◇◇◇◇◇

3 JULY 2011
The quality of tenderness

I have just seen a lovely French film, *Potiche (Trophy Wife)*, with Catherine Deneuve and Gérard Depardieu. Watching Depardieu set me thinking again about that elusive quality called tenderness. This is a quality which this strange giant of a man (and he has now become almost gross in size) shares with another large actor, Robbie Coltrane. A friend of mine commented upon this after seeing the film. 'What an attractive man Depardieu is,' she said with surprise in her voice. And I knew exactly what she meant. The tenderness shines out of his eyes, a quality of gentle loving-kindness which draws us to him. It is the eyes, those windows of our soul, which reveal the capacity of their owner's soul to express love, and, in the case of these two actors, their eyes show it so unreservedly and warmly. It is worth going to see *Potiche* just for those few moments when Depardieu looks at Deneuve with love, and also for the beautiful scene in which the two of them, both middle-aged and slightly ungainly, dance gently together. This is more erotic than many much more explicit love scenes often lacking in any tenderness whatsoever.

It is a quality we need much of as acupuncturists.

5 JULY 2011
Why are actresses called actors now?

In my last blog I wrote about a film actor and an actress, and found myself irritated yet again by the, to me, utterly ridiculous convention which appeared some years back out of nowhere, and I hope may, at some time in the future, disappear as quickly again, that of calling actresses actors. Is this political correctness gone mad? We still distinguish a husband from a wife, a girl from a boy, a widow from a widower, a prince from a princess, so why not an actor from an actress? Of course some professions only have one word in English to describe both male and female practitioners, such as a barrister or a doctor, perhaps because women were only admitted later to these professions, whilst actresses belong to a long tradition. And nobody appears to have thought of calling a female barrister a barristress or a female doctor a doctress, although this is what other languages do. But why replace a perfectly good word which has been used for centuries? And in an obscure way, I find its removal to be demeaning rather than respectful to women, as though we all need to make an effort to remember gender equality.

Interestingly, the convention has not yet crept into everyday speech, where people still talk about the actress Judi Dench, but in the written press and on radio or television it has been banished to the archives, the latter obviously by BBC edict. And yet I was amused the other day to hear a journalist stumbling over himself, the word 'actress' coming out unbidden, before being quickly corrected to 'actor'.

Can anybody tell me when and why the change from actress to actor took place?

◇◇◇◇◇◇◇◇

7 JULY 2011
Mandarin – here I come!

The translation of my *Handbook of Five Element Acupuncture* into Chinese (see my blog, *Meetings with remarkable people*, of 16 June 2011) is a moment of completion for me, as if my journey into five element acupuncture, started more than 25 years back, has now come full circle, very satisfyingly. All the fears I had for five element acupuncture as I closed my school some four years ago have, in a surprisingly different way from any that I could have imagined, proved groundless. Here now the door back to China, and with it to all those countless people who still look to China to guide them in their approach to traditional Chinese medicine, has re-opened itself to this beloved discipline of mine, and invited it back in. I feel that my work has indeed been accomplished.

But not quite yet fully! For I am invited to China once my book appears on Chinese bookshelves, and to prepare for this I feel, as a former linguist, proud of trying never to travel to a country without at least some slight knowledge of its language, that it would be discourteous of me not to learn at least the rudiments of Mandarin in order to be able to respond with some respect to what my Chinese hosts will be saying. I have always been surprised that I have delayed so long before immersing myself in the Chinese language which underpins all acupuncture in a very profound way, particularly as I am now translating Elisabeth Rochat de la Vallée's *Les 101 notions-clés de la médecine chinoise* (101 Key Concepts). Perhaps it was simply a matter of never finding the time, for I tried to start several times, or because I was afraid (and still am) that my increasingly deficient hearing will not pick up the nuances of Chinese speech. But now I intend to make up for this strange omission if I can, and am about to enrol in an intensive Mandarin course. More of this anon!

◇◇◇◇◇◇◇◇◇

10 JULY 2011
The significance of a Husband/Wife imbalance and its diagnosis

I have written this blog in answer to a query from somebody commenting on my blog of 23 June in my sister blog www.five-element-treatments.blogspot.com, but I think it is important enough to include here in this blog. I was asked how I had diagnosed a Husband/Wife imbalance just by looking at the patient. What did I observe that made me diagnose H/W? I give my answer below. It is a very detailed answer because the question encouraged me to think carefully what a H/W imbalance means, and touches upon what is a very complex and profound area, that of pulse diagnosis.

We are told to diagnose a H/W through the pulses, with the pulses of the left side, the 'husband's' side being qualitatively stronger than those of the right, 'the wife's'. Diagnosis from pulses alone presupposes that our pulse-taking is sensitive enough to feel what may be an extremely subtle difference. I have often said, and will go on repeating, that it is foolish to rely entirely on our pulse-taking in making a diagnosis, since it is a very great skill accurately to interpret what the pulses are telling us, acquired only after years of practice. To understand this, but certainly not to be too daunted by this, it is essential that we remember at all times what we are attempting to assess at those six positions at each wrist that we gently palpate to give us a pulse-reading of the 12 officials forming the five elements.

We should think of the 12 pulses as access points to the elements. They can be palpated most clearly where the blood flow is at its strongest and nearest the surface. Since time immemorial in traditional Chinese medicine, and in modern times in Western medicine, too, the most easily accessible point has been accepted as being over the radial artery at the wrist. It is important to visualize the pattern the 12 pulses form on any pulse chart, and here we should divide them into six, since at each position there are two, one at the superficial level and one at the deep level. (I know that different diagrams of the pulses have been drawn up over the centuries showing an intermediate position, which would in effect make 18 possible pulses, and also different pulse positions, particularly in relation to one of the pulses on the right side (the five element Outer Fire pulses), but I am writing here only about the order of the pulses which five element acupuncturists use.)

In effect, the understanding that the five elements will reveal the state of their health in body and soul at a tiny site like this, less than a couple of inches (oh how I still love my old form of measurement!) (a few cms) in length, is awe-inspiring and still blows my mind. It means, in effect, that the work of all the elements acting together is creating the blood flow at every point in the body, not just at the wrist, but that it can be detected most easily where the arterial blood is closest to the surface. (Pulses can also be palpated at the ankle or over the carotid artery in the neck where there are equally strong pulsations, but the wrist is used for reasons of easy access.) It is important always to remember the order of the pulses, and here not just the order on each hand but the order of both hands taken together. If we hold the hands together facing upwards (do this now if you are reading this), imagine that you are drawing a line which starts at the pulses nearest the wrist on the left hand, moves down to the two other pulse positions on the left wrist and then passes over to the pulses on the right hand, continuing down to the third position on the right before looping back over again to the first pulses of the left hand again, forming a continuous figure of eight. In effect, we are tracing the order of the elements backwards, from Inner Fire (Heart/Small Intestine), back to Wood and Water, back across to the right wrist to Metal, Earth and Outer Fire (Heart Protector/Three Heater), before looping back to the inner side of Fire again and so on.

We are taught to palpate the pulses in this way, first left-hand pulses starting with the first position over the Heart/Small Intestine aspect of Fire and then right-hand pulses starting with the Metal pulses. This is a simple way of reading the pulses, and emphasizes the importance of the Heart pulse as being the first pulse we palpate, but in doing this we tend to forget the actual order of the elements, even if we were ever aware that the pulses represent this, which many of us are not. It is only in helping us make a Husband/Wife diagnosis (and that of an Entry/Exit block) that it is so imperative to think of this order to understand what our pulses are telling us.

We know that the flow of energy moves along the Sheng cycle from Fire to Earth to Metal etc. We know also that we correct a H/W by needling the following points: III (Bl) 67, IV(Ki) 7, VIII (Liv) 4, IV (Ki) 3, II (SI) 4, I (Ht) 7. This order of points does the following: First it reconnects the mother element, Metal (a right-hand pulse) with its child, Water (a left-hand pulse), then, by needling VIII (Liv) 4, it draws energy from the Metal element (right-hand pulse) across the Ke cycle to the Wood element (mother element to grandchild element) (left-hand pulse), then by needling Ki 3 it does the same from Earth across the Ke cycle to Water, and finally it reinforces the Heart by needling the source points of Inner Fire, finishing with Ht 7.

In effect, by diagnosing an excess of energy in the right-hand pulses and a frightening depletion of energy in the left-hand pulses, the classic diagnosis of H/W, the pulses are telling us that there is a potential breakdown between the elements, and in particular between the point at which energy from Metal passes over to its child, Water. It isn't a complete breakdown, because that means death, but it is sufficiently serious for us to regard a H/W imbalance as a dangerous condition because it is depleting the energy flowing to the Heart. It is therefore interesting to see how often the pulses leap back into balance immediately Metal is reconnected more strongly to Water, i.e., after needling III (Bl) 67, IV (Ki) 7. It is therefore a good idea to read the pulses after you have needled these two points to see if you can detect the immediate sign of relief as the energy flow starts to re-establish itself, and the Heart can begin to relax.

With all this in mind, I will go back to the question which has prompted this exposition of what a H/W imbalance actually represents. If it reveals a serious weakening of the flow of energy from mother to child element around the complete cycle of the five elements, which it does, then this serious weakening must somehow show itself not only on the pulses but in the way a patient presents themselves, which it does. Patients will look despairing, as if they have given up hope (the Heart almost giving in). As well as showing this despair, they will surprisingly often say things which help our diagnosis, such as, 'I don't think I can go on' or 'I feel like giving up'. They may look as if they are too weak to talk, just wanting to lie there passive with their eyes closed.

H/W can appear suddenly, as though the Heart all at once can take no more, unlike imbalances such as Aggressive Energy which appear slowly over time, so the change in a patient from one treatment to the next can be very obvious. In the case of the patient I was writing about, he came into the room looking so very different from how he had left me the week before, that the change was dramatic enough for me to suspect H/W even before I took his pulses.

Finally, I repeat my mantra, 'Never rely on pulses alone to tell you what is going on.' Use all your senses and all your feelings and any other diagnostic information to help you diagnostically, such as a patient rubbing their eyes in the case of a II/III (SI/Bl) block or the onset of hay-fever in the case of a X/XI (LI/St) block, since our pulse-taking (mine included) may not be sensitive enough to do the diagnosis on its own.

◇◇◇◇◇◇◇◇

13 JULY 2011

There are 25 ways of expressing the five emotions

It is worth remembering that, since each of us is composed of a unique combination of all the five elements, and each element expresses every one of the five emotions, there are in effect 25 possible expressions of the different emotions. The five principal categories which tradition associates with a particular element, such as joy for Fire and fear for Water, are therefore modified when it is not a Fire person expressing joy or a Water person expressing fear. When a Metal person expresses joy or fear, those expressions of joy or fear will be shaded by grief, Metal's dominant emotion, and therefore will express themselves in a different way from a Wood person expressing joy or fear, or a Fire or Water person expressing joy or fear.

It is therefore not simply a matter of observing joy or fear expressed to their fullest in Fire or Water people, but of having experience of observing these emotions in people who are not Fire or Water. We have to begin to differentiate the type of joy or fear being shown, however much this may be buried beneath the dominant emotion of another element. Fire or Water will show these two emotions in their purest form, since they pour out straight from the organs controlled by these two elements, whereas joy shown by an Earth person or fear shown by a Metal person will be modified by the patina of sympathy or thoughtfulness Earth throws over all it does and the patina of grief which Metal shows in all it does. In other words they will show an Earth or Metal-type joy or fear, which will be quite different from joy or fear expressed in pure form by Fire or Water.

In trying to gain a foothold in the tricky world of interpreting the emotional signatures of an element, we therefore have to look carefully at all the different possible nuances of emotional expression. We have to bring to this all the knowledge of the elements we have accumulated so far to help point us in one of the five directions. We can do this in retrospect, as it were, by looking carefully at a person whose element we are sure of, and observing how they express the emotions of the other four elements, not just their own. How, for example, does a Metal person express their anger or their sympathy, or a Wood person their grief or their fear? Such an exercise is a very useful way of expanding our library of pointers to the different elements.

Unfortunately words are inadequate tools to describe such subtle distinctions, so, regretfully, this blog is the only answer I can give to the request of another acupuncturist who asked if I 'could perhaps say something about the different responses you have to the control of Wood and the control of Fire. I have a patient who is like a blazing log stack, a wonderful human in there but very controlling, and I can't come down on a CF (guardian element).' Sorry I can't help you more than this, Kate, except to encourage you to focus your emotional antennae a little more each time you see this patient. Something about the nature of what you see as his/her controlling character will eventually point you to one or other element (which may after all prove to be neither Wood nor Fire, just to confuse you further!). But give it time! We're usually, if not always, in more of a hurry than our patients.

◇◇◇◇◇◇◇◇

24 JULY 2011
Preparing to meet a new patient

I have written before about the courage it takes to be a practitioner as we prepare to confront the unknown in each new patient we meet (see my blog of 25 April 2011 on *The unknowability of another human being*). I am preparing myself to do just that this week when I meet a new patient for the first time.

It will be up to me to ensure that I conduct this meeting in such a way that it ends with my patient feeling that I have already helped her in some way. It should also leave me feeling, not that I must 'know the patient's element', as though that is the be-all and end-all of this initial interaction, but that I know enough about her to make her feel happy to come back a second time.

Of course this knowledge, and all the other little bits of knowledge I will gain each time I meet her, will eventually together point me towards one element, I hope, but even if I feel confident about the element early on, that alone will never be sufficient. Just deciding on an element, however correctly we may make our diagnosis, only does so much, unless we add to it that deeper level of understanding, that 'soul to soul' bit, which will give to our treatment its special flavour. And we must never forget that we can start off on what we eventually find is not the right element and yet help our patients at a deep level through our empathy with them.

Above all, I must be curious. Perhaps I am fortunate that I have always been fascinated by glimpses of other people's lives. If I am amongst a group of people, what I most enjoy is sitting back, unobserved, and watching how they interact with one another. These interactions are endlessly fascinating, and, for a five element acupuncturist, endlessly instructive. I must bring this curiosity with me as the most important gift I will be bringing to my new patient. I need to gather all those snippets she will tell me about her loves, her longings and her disappointments, and use them to start building up a picture of her life and how she lives it now and will hope to be living it better in the future if the treatment for which she has approached me is to help her. And then I will need to look deeply into myself and examine how what she has told me, and the way in which she told me this, points me in the direction of one element.

I have learnt over the years not to be too hard on myself, and not to allow any dissatisfaction I may feel about the way I conduct this first encounter to affect me too deeply. I can only do the best I can at the time, and if I feel that I have somehow failed my patient in some way by not quite adjusting my approach sensitively enough, then there is always the next time in which to correct this. We must never ask too much of ourselves in this very delicate business of our engagement with our patients. As long as they feel we care about them, they will always come back a next time and give us another chance to get things a little more right.

29 JULY 2011

Find the element, and the points will look after themselves

I am not somebody who enjoys experimenting in my acupuncture. I regard myself as a steady plodder, and like to think I work my way along paths well-trodden before me. One of the ways in which this somewhat cautious approach reveals itself is in my choice of points. I have often said that I have a very small repertoire of points, concentrating mainly on those few points which have a close and safe relationship with the element I am treating. I focus mostly on the command points, then on other points on the elements which I have gathered together over the years, on points which release energy blocks of all kinds, and finally, and only then, on that difficult but important category of points which we select, as we say, 'for their spirit'. It is this group which causes every acupuncturist the most trouble, since it is like opening a can of worms, as we ask ourselves which point exactly we need to use for its spirit for this particular patient on this particular day, and often can't come up with the answer.

What I don't usually do, though, is experiment. I have not had the habit, as other acupuncturists apparently have, of looking up the list of acupuncture points and branching out in a new direction by choosing a point I have never used, usually basing this choice on a point's name. I have thought about this quite a lot recently, because I am at the stage in my practice where I am enjoying injecting something new into it, and what can be newer than using a point I have never used before? So, venturing on to new terrain, I have done this for one or two patients and then stood back to assess whether

I have learnt anything from this experiment, and whether, more crucially, my patients, thus experimented upon, have responded in ways that differ from their responses to the more familiar kinds of treatment I have offered them before.

What I find, not unexpectedly, is that I really could not say what effect any of these new points have had, except that, as usual, my patients have continued to improve as they did before with my familiar array of points. I asked myself whether there was any sign that something new had occurred, and came up with the answer, 'no'. So on a very small sample of just a few treatments, certainly, a mathematician would say, not a statistically significant number of any kind, I learnt nothing which shook my long-held belief that the fundamental nature of any five element treatment consists in addressing the element, rather than worrying about the points we use to address this element. I will always stick to my mantra, 'Think element, not points,' to help me in my practice. The selection of points then always becomes secondary to the importance of selecting the right element.

So take heart all those many acupuncturists who seem to worry too much about point selection, and particularly about what exactly 'selecting points for their spirit' means. All points, particularly those all-important command points, have a 'spirit'.

Once you find the element, the points will look after themselves.

Much of what I like to write about concerns the subtleties of human relationships, and how these act themselves out in our relationship with our patients. This blog is another one which emphasizes how slight alterations in the way we frame our questions can close a patient down completely or allow them the freedom to open up to us if they want to.

◇◇◇◇◇◇◇◇◇

2 AUGUST 2011

The art of asking the right questions in the right way

Since seeing a new patient for the first time last week I have been thinking a lot about what is the right and what the wrong way of saying things. Twice I found myself asking a question awkwardly or saying something clumsily, but realized this in time, and quietly re-phrased what I was saying in a way that satisfied me.

The first time was when I asked my patient, 'Are you happy with your life?', and realized immediately that this was not the right way to frame the question. I then changed it quickly to, 'How happy are you with your life?' Thinking back on this, I realize that my initial question gave my patient only the option of saying 'yes' or 'no', either reply being unlikely to reflect the truth, since nobody is either truly only happy or only unhappy about all aspects of their life. Such a black and white question makes it easy only to respond with a black and white reply, leaving no room for all those grey areas in which we live our lives most of the time, sometimes happy, sometimes unhappy, but never either of these all the time.

The second time was when my patient told me that she was going back to Ireland to see her family for the first time in four years, and I found the words 'How lovely! How exciting for you!' coming to my lips, before I bit them off in time, and asked instead, 'Are you looking forward to this or are you dreading it?' My first question was like one of those meaningless interchanges we litter our social life with and which mean absolutely nothing, such as, 'How are you?', 'I'm fine'. It would effectively have closed the door on any hope of hearing how my patient actually felt about seeing her family after such a long time. Why had she left it so long, after all, if it was a good relationship? Ireland, unlike Australia, is easy to travel to.

On such little shifts in the way we frame our questions and responses to our patients often hangs the development of a good or tricky relationship with our patients. I still myself remember the time when a friend told me that she was surprised that I had reacted as I did to something that had happened, and said, 'I can't understand why you didn't...' That effectively stopped me from telling her anything more about myself, because I felt I was regarded as a bit odd for being as I was. Instead of being offered an implied criticism, what I would have responded well to would have been to have been asked why I did what I did.

And we must make sure that our engagement with our patients, too, gives them the freedom to tell us truly why they did what they did and felt what they felt. We must never assume we know the answers to this. Only our patient does.

◇◇◇◇◇◇◇◇

3 AUGUST 2011
We can only cope with what we can cope with

As I get older, I hope I get a little wiser and also a little more tolerant of my own inadequacies. And one of the snippets of wisdom this year has taught me is contained in a mantra I now say to myself, 'We can only cope with what we can cope with.' It's no good our being cross at ourselves or at others for doing things which, at the time or with the benefit of hindsight, we know are not wise things to do or to have done. It is difficult enough working our way through the stresses life presents us with without adding to them the weight of too much guilt when we feel that our actions have been misguided. I think it is therefore good to get used to telling ourselves that that is all we could have done at the time.

It is a particularly useful lesson for me as a five element acupuncturist, because understanding what any particular patient can cope with is another one of the subtle ways of tracing the imprint of an element. When we realize, for example, that Metal cannot cope with the sort of things Fire can, or Wood with what Earth can, we are on our way to understanding a little better what makes the different elements tick.

My blogs area interspersed with references to my contact with Liu Lihong in China, and the stimulation my own work dedicated to promote five element acupuncture has gained from the vast new world being opened to me over there. I have always regretted the need to close my school, the School of Five Element Acupuncture (SOFEA) in 2007, but never disputed the fact that this was the right decision. I have always been sensitive to changes in the air surrounding the future of acupuncture and those which heralded the financial crisis of 2008 and the forced closure of two traditional acupuncture colleges. I could see the writing on the wall for small independent acupuncture colleges in the UK. I therefore decided the time was right to stop my next intake of students, complete the training of all the current students who had enrolled with us, and sadly close the school's doors.

With hindsight this decision was the only right one in the financial climate of the time, but it opened up what could have been a void in my life, depriving me of the possibility of guiding others in the ways of five element acupuncture. Not so, it turned out, and, as Liu Lihong told me one day in Nanning, 'You see,

Nora, closing your school made it possible for you to come to China.' And as the saying goes, as one door closes, another opens. Looking at things now, some few years after writing this blog in 2011, I can see the truth of what he told me. I could not have found the time to do what I am now doing in China if I were still engrossed in all the day-to-day activities of running an acupuncture college in England.

◇◇◇◇◇◇◇◇

14 AUGUST 2011
Now China, here I come!

Everybody interested in the future of five element acupuncture will share my delight that it is now making its way back to China, carried first on the wings of the Chinese-language edition of my *Handbook of Five Element Acupuncture*, which will be in Chinese bookshops in a week or so, and then by my own presence in China. I have been invited over there at the end of October by Liu Lihong of the Clinical Research Institute of Classical Chinese Medicine attached to the Guangxi College of Traditional Chinese Medicine. He is a colleague of Heiner Fruehauf, who many of you will know as the author of the very important article 'Chinese Medicine in Crisis' (*Journal of Chinese Medicine* No 61, October 1999). You can also see Liu Lihong talking to Heiner on the website www.ClassicalChineseMedicine.org. He encouraged Mei Long, a Chinese postgraduate student of mine, now living in the Netherlands, to translate the *Handbook*.

I will be flying first to Chengdu, then to the Guanxi College of Traditional Chinese Medicine in Nanning to teach a group of acupuncturists there for about a week. I will then fly on to Beijing to give a seminar at the large international conference which Liu Lihong is organizing. He regards this as a very significant step in the important programme of re-introducing five element acupuncture to China and re-attaching Chinese acupuncture more firmly to its traditional roots. (Heiner's article is a very good introduction to the background to this.)

It is a great honour to have been invited by him and to have been recognized by him as an important contributor to his work.

More blogs about my visit on my return from China.

◇◇◇◇◇◇◇◇

15 AUGUST 2011

An illuminating article by Heiner Fruehauf all should read

I have just read Heiner's article on 'Chinese Medicine in Crisis: Science, Politics, and the Making of "TCM"', which appears in the August 2011 newsletter of his website www. ClassicalchineseMedicine.org.

I give below the quotation from Li Zhichong, Director of the Chinese TCM Association, 2002, with which he heads his article:

'The latter half of the 19th century and through the end of the 20th century has been a time of great political, economic, cultural, and scientific transformation in China. Chinese medicine, the shining gem of traditional science, has had to endure many assaults in this process, sinking the field into a quagmire where it had to fight bitterly for its own survival. This course of events can be called "The Century when Traditional Chinese Medicine was Tied up in the Straitjacket of Utter Delusion".'

Heiner writes that his article 'is based on the conviction that the traditional art of Oriental medicine is dying – both in mainland China, home of the mother trunk of the field, and consequently overseas where branches of the tree are trying to grow.'

I think everybody who wants to gain a deeper understanding of the current state of traditional Chinese medicine throughout the world will find something to ponder about in this article.

◇◇◇◇◇◇◇◇

29 AUGUST 2011
The energy of Fire

In the past few weeks I have become very aware of the Fire element, particularly as here in England we hardly seem to have had a summer before late summer is in the air, and even, oh horror, so early, a hint of the autumn to come. Perhaps my own Fire element has craved more of the warmth and sunlight it needs to fill it before its season passes, but, whatever the reason, it is at Fire that I find that I am looking with somewhat new eyes.

For what I have noticed increasingly, in a way that I did not do before, is the sheer energy this element shows in all it does, like a spring within it always coiled and ready to be released at each new encounter with the world. It is even there in its smile, an outpouring of warmth towards others, very unlike the timid, passive or more withdrawn smiles of other elements. I don't think I had realized until now quite how much yang energy is contained in this most yang of all elements, whose season, after all is high summer, the yang high-point of the year.

I think we often regard Fire as being a gentle element, perhaps because we believe that the love that it brings to bear on all things is a gentle emotion, which it so rarely is, just as Fire is far from being as gentle as the impression it likes to give of itself. I have recently been looking at videos on YouTube of famous Chinese people to take as examples close to home for when I teach in China, and this is when I was struck, so unexpectedly, by the weight of energy pouring out in all Fire's movements. Watching yet again the Chinese pianist, Lang Lang, it is so vividly clear in the way he plays. Through his playing he reaches out forcefully to the conductor in front of him, the orchestra around him and the audience beyond him, almost as though trying to capture them with his joy. I compared this with other pianists I know, some of whom will sit quite still and withdrawn at the piano, so yin-like, as though communing silently with the music and apparently, during these moments of their playing, unaware of the world beyond them.

So if you are a five element acupuncturist and are trying to work out ways of recognizing Fire, watch out for the energy you feel coming towards you. And then learn to compare this with the very different energies of those other two powerful elements, Wood and Water. Wood does not try to share anything with you in the way Fire so ardently would like to do, but wants more to force itself on to you. Water's energetic thrust is much more elusive, being apparently so gentle at one moment, and then, like flood water, sweeping you aside in its rush to survive.

I am always delighted to discover yet again the elements' ability to surprise me with the variety of ways in which they reveal their differences.

◇◇◇◇◇◇◇◇

13 SEPTEMBER 2011
Losing control in the practice room

I am still surprised at how easily I can allow myself to be controlled by a patient even after all these years of practice. This may come from my desire to please others (my Fire wanting everybody around them to be happy), which can lead me too quickly to do something which I don't really want to do and which I eventually realize is not right for me to do. My Small Intestine is also always only too ready to think that the other person may be right in what they are demanding of me, and it is only after some thought that I may decide that this is not so, by which time I may well have agreed to something I eventually come to regret.

In the practice situation this may reveal itself as not being quick enough to realize that in some way I am being manipulated by a patient, something as practitioners we all know can happen when patients, who may feel uneasy about coming for treatment, try to wrench control back into their own hands. This may appear as something apparently so insignificant as a patient who has already undergone major intrusive surgical procedures making an extreme fuss about the heat of a tiny moxa cone, or a determination not to accept a practitioner's time constraints.

This is what happened today. A new patient, very uneasy indeed from the moment he walked in the door, managed to get me to make the next appointment on a day which I had crossed out in my diary with the words 'Keep day free' written in big letters across it. It was only after he had gone that I realized what had happened, as I tried to analyze the great feeling of disempowerment which his treatment had left me with. Though I was cross at myself for allowing myself to be outmanoeuvred in this way, I had to laugh because, feeling as I did that his element was Water, it had, as usual, managed to get its own way, and I, as Fire, had, as usual, allowed myself temporarily to be extinguished by its force.

Obviously each element will offer different challenges to different practitioners, and practitioners who are not Fire may not recognize this particular challenge, but everybody should look carefully at which situations cause them the greatest stress and then try to trace this back to the element or elements in their patients which are causing this. It is also an excellent way of helping ourselves track down an element, as I found in this instance. My careful unravelling of why this patient had made me uneasy helped to strengthen my belief that I was dealing here with Water.

Now my task is to try to regain control at the next treatment, and to make sure that my Fire blazes sufficiently strongly to turn the powerful force of his Water into less threatening steam. A good lesson for me, and I hope for anybody else reading this who has found themselves struggling to remain in control in the practice room. And the moment we lose control, we also lose our ability to help.

<><><><><><><>

29 SEPTEMBER 2011
One of a practitioner's greatest qualities must be curiosity

I was reminded yesterday of one of the most important qualities a good five element practitioner needs to possess, and if they do not already possess it, needs to cultivate as thoroughly as possible, and that is curiosity, pure and simple – curiosity, put baldly, about what makes us ourselves and those around us tick.

The particular incident from yesterday's practice which made me think about this came about when I was called in by another practitioner to look at a patient of hers, 'whom', as she put it, 'I can't quite get a handle on.' She felt that the patient was holding her at arms' length all the time, and wondered if she was not treating the right element, which she had, in my opinion rightly, diagnosed as Fire. I could feel that though the patient was friendly, pleasant and smiling all the time, she was indeed keeping the deep part of herself firmly locked away from us.

Why was this? And what had happened that had made her so defensive? There was something here to explore, and our diagnosis of her element helped me find a way in. Fire wants above all to relate. It needs relationships, particularly sexual relationships, in the way that Earth needs to be nourished and Metal craves self-respect. She had not been in a long-term relationship for many years, because 'I always choose the wrong person.' I decided to address this issue head-on and asked, 'Did any relationship you have had in the past end by breaking your heart?', and was not surprised to hear that, yes, one had. Her first really deep relationship had lasted three years and should have ended in marriage if she had not discovered very close to the wedding day that he was a serial philanderer. Living as she did in a very small, tightly knit community, she was then forced to be a witness to his marrying a friend of hers with whom he now has several children.

It was interesting to watch the change in this patient as she talked about all this. There was obviously relief at being able to tell us her story, and a great deal of sadness as she did so, but also, after a lovely further treatment on Fire, starting with IV (Ki) 24, Spirit Burial Ground to resuscitate her damaged spirit, a kind of transformation within her as her Fire element started to heal itself at a deep level and no longer needed to throw up such a defensive screen around to protect her.

This was a lovely treatment with a lovely result, and a lesson to us all to persist in our questioning until we get to the core of a patient's troubles. And I only really managed to reach this core when my persistent but gentle questioning at last got through her defences and made her feel safe enough to say what in effect she had held back from saying for years. Interestingly, patients themselves are often unaware of the long-term effects of something that happened years ago upon the present state of their health, as this patient was. This patient's ostensible reason for coming for treatment was not the hurt this failed relationship had inflicted upon her, but a physical complaint, persistent headaches. It was only my questioning that gradually revealed to her the true depth of the pain this first love of her life had inflicted upon her.

Here the element we choose will guide us in the type of questioning we need to pursue. If she had been Metal, for example, I would perhaps not have focused so much on relationships but upon the areas of her life which had brought her the greatest sense of self-fulfilment. It is not enough, then, simply to say that the patient is Fire or Metal. We have to know exactly what kind of things have happened to force that Fire or Metal so far out of shape that it can no longer function properly. And we are only able to find this out by being really curious to know what has gone on in our patient's life and by not being afraid to tackle deep areas of hurt. I sometimes feel I go 'where angels fear to tread', but that angels are there to beckon me in.

9 OCTOBER 2011

Regaining control in the practice room: how the elements cast their magic upon patient and practitioner

This blog is a follow-up to my blog of 13 September 2011 on *Losing control in the practice room.*

I am delighted to be able to say that this patient's next treatment not only restored my faith in my own ability to maintain control, but also, and, far more importantly, showed me once again how the elements cast their magic not only upon our patients as they start to heal them, but also upon us as practitioners, as they remind us of their ability to transform.

My patient appeared at the door of my practice room as, in my eyes, quite another person. He greeted me less nervously, and with a warm smile that had not been there last time. He was much less nervous of the needles, chatted about his week's work very easily, and interestingly did not, as he had done last time, demand a time for his next appointment. Instead, he apologized that his work-schedule was making it difficult for me to fit him into the times I normally see patients. The relationship between us had relaxed markedly. I can only attribute this to the transformative effect, on my patient, of strengthening his Water element and thus reducing his fear, and, on me, of helping me understand that the somewhat threatening interplay between us at his first treatment was caused by his fear and by my not responding appropriately to this fear.

And so I continue to learn.

◇◇◇◇◇◇◇◇

19 OCTOBER 2011

The dangers facing traditional Chinese medicine

I am preparing what I want to say about five element acupuncture on my visit to China, and am finding the process surprisingly challenging. After years of talking about my love for what I do, how exactly do I want to convey this love to a new audience, and an audience, above all, whose understanding of the elements is so very deep-rooted that I hesitate to think that I have anything new to add to what they already know?

And then today, to help me in my search for the right words, I came across a fascinating video of a Chinese master of traditional medicine discussing the problems he sees confronting it today, and this gave me the lead I needed. He talked about the 'standardization process' to which it is being subjected in China, and which, he says, is leading to a 'thinning out of the depth of Chinese medicine'. The evocative phrase 'thinning out' resonated with me, and goes right to the heart of what I think is happening not only in China but throughout the world; it has become a process of etiolation. This is a lovely word I have often longed to use, and which leapt to my mind as such words do as I write. The dictionary defines it as 'making plants pale by excluding light' and 'giving a sickly hue'. I think this is a vivid and true description of how I view the dangers facing traditional Chinese medicine everywhere, including in its birthplace, China, and which threaten to drain it of much of its vitality.

So off I fly next week to add what I hope is my own little bit of bright colour and light to what is taught over there!

◇◇◇◇◇◇◇◇◇

25 OCTOBER 2011
Finally off to China!

This is my last blog before I am off to China, and then there will be a silence from me for three weeks into which will pour all the impressions awaiting me there – impressions not only of the vast country and its people, but of what I foresee as being an awesome moment, as I touch the spirit of the place from whose roots what I do sprung more than two thousand years ago.

I like to see myself and all those practising five element acupuncture each as a tiny bud upon one of the branches of the mighty tree of acupuncture. I know that my own bud will be nourished by visiting its ancient homeland, and I hope in turn that my visit will add a little bit more nourishment to its roots.

I am busily rehearsing the few lines of greeting in Mandarin with which I hope to start my seminars both in Nanning and in Beijing, but I am not holding myself to saying them if my courage fails me at the last moment and I find myself reverting to the safety of English!

I look forward to reporting back in future blogs on my return.

◇◇◇◇◇◇◇◇◇

16 NOVEMBER 2011

My first blog about my visit to China (written on the Great Wall on Sunday 13 November before leaving for home)

What can I say? I'm sitting on the Great Wall in China trying to catch my breath, both physically, because of the steep steps leading to it, and emotionally, because of all that has gone on since our arrival two weeks ago. I am also trying to fit what we did into bite-sized packets of information, and then into words suitable for my blog.

All I can now say is that it has been in every way a totally moving, instructive, warm and overwhelmingly fruitful experience, with ramifications for five element acupuncture which spread out to the furthest corners of China, to which the 500 or so seminar participants who came to Beijing to listen to me are now returning, with new thoughts about what is, to them, an utterly new approach to acupuncture to mull over.

More, much more, when I have had time to collect my thoughts after my return to London the day after tomorrow.

◇◇◇◇◇◇◇◇◇

20 NOVEMBER 2011

A refreshingly new acupuncture landscape

There was something very stimulating about moving from what I have come to regard as the somewhat weary world of acupuncture in the UK to a refreshingly new acupuncture landscape in China. The wonder of this whole experience was that I was speaking to people to whom the world of the elements is a familiar place, unlike those first embarking on acupuncture in the West, and who therefore had such a quick understanding of the principles of five element acupuncture, and only needed to be given a few signposts to guide them.

The most concentrated teaching was in Nanning, in Guanxi province in the south, where I taught at a newly opened centre for traditional medicine, the Tong You San He, founded by Professor Liu Lihong at whose invitation I was in China. On most days the group consisted of up to 50 people, of whom about 15 are serious students of five element acupuncture.

Then after nine long days of teaching, which included the treatment of many people, both privately and in front of the class, we had two days' relaxing time travelling to the Guilin Mountains and up the Li River to Yangshou. I was very moved to see at last the very mountains whose photo I had chosen as the front cover of my *Handbook* many years before. Again something coming full circle.

Then on up north to Beijing and to a large traditional medicine conference at which I spoke to the 500 or so participants, each of whom, flatteringly, was holding a copy of the Mandarin version of my *Handbook*, which they had been given in their conference bags. After the seminar, much signing of books and much taking of photos.

The response wherever I taught was overwhelming, with people asking again and again, 'Where can we learn five element acupuncture?' Where indeed! It has proved difficult enough in the UK over the years to find good five element teaching, and over there it will be even more difficult. But being such an enterprising nation, I have no doubt that they will find a way. And I like to think that I will continue to be there to accompany those amongst them who wish to set their feet ever more firmly on the five element path.

This is the point at which I started to think about the need to write something in the nature of a Self-Tuition Manual for my Chinese students, since it was obvious that there would never be sufficient five element teachers to satisfy the growing need of China's acupuncturists to retrieve the roots of the more spiritual approach to acupuncture which they have glimpsed in five element acupuncture. This then gradually turned into various drafts for the Teach Yourself Manual which is now included as an Appendix in the much-revised version of my *Handbook of Five Element Practice*.

◇◇◇◇◇◇◇◇◇

25 NOVEMBER 2011
Where do we go from here?

There were so many people asking where they could learn more about five element acupuncture in China that I must now think carefully what will be the best way to go forward from here, and build upon this exciting new ground.

There is already a small band of about 15 students in Nanning who will form the nucleus of a five element school in the future, and we must concentrate on helping them learn more. The challenging part will be to work out a programme of teaching which takes account of the different levels of expertise of this group. How much they will learn and how quickly they will feel confident enough to incorporate five element acupuncture into their practice will depend to a great extent upon how well I structure the different levels of teaching required.

A lot of hard work lies ahead but it represents an exciting new challenge for me.

◇◇◇◇◇◇◇◇◇

3 DECEMBER 2011

A simple guide to five element treatments

It is with the encouragement of my good friend, Peter Eckman, the author of *In the Footsteps of the Yellow Emperor* (still in my view the best, if not the only, detailed history of acupuncture's migration from East to West), that I have started to think about writing a book about the first few treatments any five element acupuncturist should be considering for a new patient. I was at first a bit reluctant to do so, because it seemed to me to be a little superfluous. Surely, I thought to myself, everybody who practises five element acupuncture knows that we always start as simply as possible, directing all our attention at the element we have chosen, the one I call the guardian element, to see whether it responds to this focused attention. But to my surprise and dismay, though this may have been true of all who learnt in the good old days when JR held sway at his college in Leamington, it now most certainly is not, as I experience each time I teach a class of newly qualified acupuncturists.

I see instead people who are often confused, as we certainly were not, as to where to direct their attention. So many of them, to my despair, have been seduced into thinking that they somehow need to add to this pure approach all sorts of other things which have infiltrated into the teaching of five element acupuncture, the most harmful of all, in my opinion, being the, to me, odd idea that into the five element mix must be thrown a goodly dab of TCM to leaven it, with its quite different approach to the elements. So both the elements in the patient and the practitioners themselves doing this have become muddled as to where exactly the focus of their treatment should lie, with the resultant confusion which I witness when these practitioners ask me for help.

So whereas years ago there was no need for such a book, because so firmly entrenched in all us five element acupuncturists was a simple, focused approach to the first stages of treatment, now there appears to be a great need for somebody to disentangle what has become a confused area of practice, and lay down again the beautifully simple principle which guides each day of my practice: 'Just treat the element, and let the element tell you by its response whether you are focusing your treatment upon the right segment of the five element circle.'

So I am starting today, amongst all the other projects I am working on (a reprint of my *Keepers of the Soul* before the copies run out, my translation of Elisabeth Rochat de la Vallée's *101 Key Concepts of Chinese Medicine*, and my latest project, drawing up a distance-learning schedule for my Chinese students), to write down in a clear, not to be misunderstood way, for each element, the simple first steps every five element acupuncturist should take when treating a new patient. It pleases me, of course, that this will also be perfect for my teaching in China.

◇◇◇◇◇◇◇◇

12 DECEMBER 2011

Developing a format for five element distance-learning for my Chinese students

It is fascinating working out a distance-learning schedule for my Chinese students, because they start from a totally different position from European students. First of all, they already have a much deeper understanding of the elements as though these are etched into their bones and in their heart. The elements are companions with which they have grown up, not the rather strange aspects of life which European students have gradually to be introduced to. And then the students are very well-trained, drilled almost, in their point location and practical techniques, such as needling. So I found that I started at a higher level in terms of their practical skills.

On the other hand, they are at a much lower level in terms of much that we take for granted here in five element practice in the West, and that is in relation to a practitioner's approach to their patients. The one thing I was constantly surprised at was to hear Liu Lihong emphasizing throughout my days of teaching in Nanning what he called my compassion to the many patients I was asked to treat. When I looked at what I was doing, I realized that what, to me, is the most fundamental aspect of my practice, my warm relationship to my patients and the importance I place on establishing this from my first contact with them, was a completely new area of practice to those observing me in China. This is, after all, the essence of what we, as five element acupuncturists, are trying to do, which is to develop such a close relationship with our patients that they feel secure enough in our presence gradually to lay aside their masks and allow their elements to reveal themselves in their true colours.

So one of the first lessons I will be thinking about is to encourage the students to use even such basic skills as pulse-taking as a first step to developing the proper physical contact with their patients without which no subsequent treatment will be successful. This is why I don't agree with taking pulses with only one hand. We need both our hands to enfold the patient's hand in a warm, loving clasp. And as we feel each pulse, we should remember JR's lovely phrase as he told us how we should take pulses: 'As you feel each pulse, you are asking, "Small Intestine, how are you today? Heart, how are you today?"' If you say this to yourself, there is no way your pulse-taking can become the automatic snatching at the mere beat of a pulse which a Western pulse diagnosis has sadly turned into.

My first lesson is already winging its way to China by email. It is on the Wood element, and how the students can find ways of observing its manifestations through looking at examples of some of the patients treated in front of the class when I was there, and adding to these some famous examples of Chinese people from the Web. I have also asked them to learn the points not only according to their Chinese names, which gives each name an individual importance, but more in terms of their relationship one to another along a meridian. The point numbers we use, such as XI (St) 1–45, draw the points together and attach them more closely to the line of the meridians they lie upon, something TCM is not so concerned with.

I have also decided, to my profound delight, to use the Roman numbers for the officials, I for Heart up to XII for Spleen, which were embedded in Leamington's teaching when I was a student there, and have so unhappily and so unnecessarily been discarded for the TCM approach which likes to start instead at the Lung. (If you look at the texts upon which the original teachings coming to the UK in the 1950s were based, you will see that the Heart always appears first.) Maybe the reason the Heart has been demoted to a subsidiary position in this way reflects the lack of heart in TCM practice, something which is reflected in Liu Lihong's desire to instil more heart in his students' practice by inviting me, a Fire person (and Inner Fire as well!) to warm up the teaching for his students. He told his class several times that 'we need more Fire here'.

So Heart once again takes what I consider to be its proper place as the head, the emperor, of all the elements. Luckily the Chinese students told me that they are already familiar with Roman numerals, unlike many of my former students, which makes their task easier.

So on to Lesson 2, the Fire element, and a discussion of the importance of touch.

◇◇◇◇◇◇◇◇

15 DECEMBER 2011
I am formed from an exploding star

Amidst all the gloom in today's world, I came across this heartening bit of news in the *Guardian* today that made me smile. It was in an article entitled 'In the beginning... Supernova produces life's elements', about the explosion of a star far out in space.

'Understanding how these giant explosions create and mix materials is important because supernovae are where we get most of the elements that make up the Earth and even our own bodies. For instance, these supernovae are a major source of iron in the universe. "So we are all made of bits of exploding stars," said Mark Sullivan of Oxford University.'

I like the thought that I am made of a bit of an exploding star.

◇◇◇◇◇◇◇◇

28 DECEMBER 2011
Just a bowl of medicine soup?

I am grateful to one of my Nanning students for the following, acute observation about the challenges facing those who work in busy acupuncture clinics where they are asked to treat many patients, and who want in some way to move on to treat with five element acupuncture. Her email has prompted me to think carefully how I can help my students over in China to make the transition to five element acupuncture without endangering their livelihoods.

'With five element acupuncture I could only see four to five patients in any half-day, and with today's demand on outpatient service, this is far too little, and I will never be able to treat all the patients... I need to see about 28 patients in half a day.'

And then she goes on to say: 'However I see that in this way we are seeing a lot more patients, but we can only treat the very surface of their problems. We have not got the time to trace or to understand where their problems have actually come from. In the times we are living in now especially, people are carrying around huge emotional burdens, and their physical problems are often caused by these internal problems. We really ought to be giving our patients not just a bowl of medicine soup, but we should also find a way to give them some spiritual nourishment.'

It is quite understandable that practitioners who may work in a system based on the need to treat a lot of people as quickly as possible find it difficult to move to five element acupuncture, where we accentuate the need to develop a long-standing one-to-one relationship with our patients. These two approaches to practice, the one, the 'bowl of medicine soup' approach, and the other the 'spiritual nourishment' approach, appear to be irreconcilable, but I do not think they are. There are certainly ways of adapting what I do in my everyday London practice to what is needed in a busy outpatients' clinic, as some of my fellow practitioners have proved when they worked in the stressful conditions in Sri Lanka after the floods treating as many patients as my Nanning student is asked to treat. It is now my task to work out the best way to help my students adapt their practice.

In this context, I find it interesting that my translation work on Elisabeth Rochat de la Vallée's *101 Key Concepts of Chinese Medicine* has strengthened my understanding that the 'bowls of medicine soup' of the original pioneers of acupuncture, some 2000 years ago, contained as their most important ingredient that of 'spiritual nourishment'. The two, the physical and the spiritual, were always regarded as an indissoluble whole. The sad thing is that this has got so thoroughly lost in modern TCM, and particularly in those places where living conditions demand a high turnover of patients. It is as though patients' spirits have become irrelevant to the restoration of health. It is little wonder, then, that my Chinese students are amazed at the speed of improvement when using five element acupuncture as compared with their current acupuncture practices.

2012 BLOGS

Because of my understanding of how the five elements shape the whole of life, they provide endlessly fascinating insights into all human behaviour, forming the foundation for these blogs. Despite my initial concern that my interest in writing my blog would gradually dry up, I will probably only draw my blog to a close when I grow weary of my interest in my fellow human beings, and at this moment I cannot envisage a time when this will be.

vii

◇◇◇◇◇◇◇◇

5 JANUARY 2012

Why it is never wise to treat our friends

I have recently been asked to treat two friends, one very close and the other more a friend of a friend. Both of them were reluctant to go to another acupuncturist, and both were in quite a lot of distress.

This has made me think carefully about what has always guided me in my decision to treat or not to treat a friend. Ideally, as we all know, we should not be treating family and friends because their very closeness means that we are not detached enough to see them clearly and to cope with finding out exactly what is wrong with them. We assume, usually very wrongly, that we really know all about them, and can therefore skip doing a proper diagnosis and move straight on to treatment. But my experiences in the past have put a lie to this, for I have often assumed somebody I know is of one element and decided quite some time later that they reveal another side to themselves and I have had to change my mind. This has happened to me with a very close relative and a very close friend, both of whom I had somehow put into an element box which, looking back, I suppose I felt was part of my comfort zone. When I later discovered how wrong I had been, I realized that I had almost deliberately been overlooking aspects of these two people which made me feel uneasy. Since learning these two difficult lessons, I have been very reluctant indeed to treat those close to me, unless there is absolutely no alternative (for example, if geographically there is no other practitioner near enough to treat them, or they are hospitalized and would simply go without treatment).

With family members, however unwise being their practitioner is, it is unlikely that my treating them is going to cause a change in our relationship. With friends, I have found, things are quite different, and my relationship to the friends I have had to treat in the past has always changed, and never for the better. Usually what has happened is that the friend now views me only as their therapist, and wishes me to continue in this role even when I am not treating (by talking over symptoms or the effects of treatment in a social context, for example). In a more extreme case, the friendship itself became endangered by the fact that a somewhat competitive friend did not like to feel that I was somehow gaining the upper hand, and persisted in claiming that treatment was making her feel worse. In the end, I lost her both as friend and patient, because we never rediscovered our easy relationship of before.

In the two examples that have come my way now, I have, with a sense of relief, passed both the friend and the friend of a friend on to a fellow practitioner, knowing that I was doing the right thing. This was not done without a slight tussle, because my first impulse is to offer help to anybody asking me for help, and it requires some strength of character for me to move aside.

◇◇◇◇◇◇◇◇◇

5 JANUARY 2012

'Living on the knife-edge of insecurity'

I just sat down for a quiet moment, and casually picked up today's *Guardian*. The actress Siân Phillips was being interviewed, and in answer to the question, 'What's the best advice anyone ever gave you?', she said: 'Saunders Lewis, the great Welsh poet, befriended me. When I went to London and gave up my life in Wales, he wrote me a letter that said, "You have to live on the knife-edge of insecurity." And I thought: "OK, that's what I'll do."'

I love the phrase, 'living on the knife-edge of insecurity'. It encapsulates what I see as the need willingly to accept the often frightening challenges life presents us with.

◇◇◇◇◇◇◇◇◇

8 JANUARY 2012

A few simple tips to make a five element acupuncturist's life easier

Don't hurry! Don't worry!

The first rule is to have compassion for your patient. Compassion means to 'feel with'. The more you can feel what your patient is feeling, and therefore can understand them, the more quickly you will be able to discover which element is directing their life. Unless we allow our own hearts to resonate with our patient's feelings, we will never understand which of the five elements guides their lives.

Do not be in a hurry to diagnose the right element! The elements will wait for you to find them, and show their faces more and more clearly with time. And all elements will enjoy the kind of focused attention they receive from simple command-point-level treatments.

If you are not in a hurry, you can relax and learn to get to know your patient better. All of this will give you time to observe whether there has been any change from treatment, and show you whether or not you should continue treating that particular element.

Don't think that your patient is necessarily expecting a quick fix. Patients appreciate the care and deep concern their practitioner shows them, and return again and again for that. This is usually unexpected and rare, compared with the impersonality of doctors' surgeries and hospital waiting rooms. Patients are usually only too happy to give the practitioner all the time they need.

The most important aspect of any treatment is not the amount of time spent on the actual physical procedures, but the time it gives you to understand your patient, observe them and help them get used to you. Patients won't be counting up how many points you needle, but they will be assessing how interested you are in them and how concerned you are about them.

Think of each treatment as asking a question of the elements. The practitioner's task is to try to interpret the answers the elements give.

Do at least four treatments on any element you choose. If you are treating once a week, then this gives you at least three weeks in which to observe an element's responses.

Don't confuse the elements by changing from one element to another after only a short time or in the same treatment, if you are not sure which element you should be treating.

Don't judge any change in your patient simply by using the criteria of changes to physical complaints. Get used to assessing change in the patient as a whole, particularly in the patient's spirit and emotional balance. It is by getting better at noticing what can be even very small changes in a patient's behaviour or physical appearance that we begin to see whether our treatment is directed at the right element.

If in doubt, simplify, and do the least number of points possible. Don't judge the success of treatment by the number of points you needle. If you aren't sure where you are going with your treatment, don't add to your confusion by haphazardly piling point upon point. Try to clear your mind by just doing one pair of command points, preferably the source points. This helps you focus your attention directly and deeply upon an element. Then let the elements answer you.

Don't spend too long trying to diagnose the major blocks (Possession, Husband/Wife). They are much more difficult to diagnose than you may think. It doesn't matter if you miss them to start with. They become more and more obvious the longer they remain untreated. An expert practitioner may see them straightaway; a less experienced practitioner will inevitably take longer to recognize them. There is a risk that a newly qualified practitioner will over-diagnose blocks because of the excitement of doing them!

◇◇◇◇◇◇◇◇◇

12 JANUARY 2012
'Look up at the stars not down at your feet'

I love this quote from a speech by Stephen Hawking. I think we all spend too long looking down at our feet, whilst the stars and universe beyond are beckoning to us to look up.

After a long last blog, I'm sure you will be pleased to read this very short, and, I think, very pertinent one.

◇◇◇◇◇◇◇◇◇

29 JANUARY 2012
My mantra of the moment

The secret to understanding another person's guardian element lies hidden deep within ourselves. If we can interpret correctly how another person makes us feel, then we are on the way to understanding the dominant element which guides their life.

6 FEBRUARY 2012

Looking for different elements in people on radio and TV

Because of all the problems the UK is facing, I have been listening to a lot of radio and watching a lot of TV recently. To lighten my mood amongst all the gloom I have been amusing myself with trying to work out whether there is any correlation between a particular element and the kinds of work those I am listening to or watching do.

Foremost amongst the people I have looked at are journalists who report the news. You would imagine that a certain kind of journalist who becomes a newscaster is there to present the human face of the news, and would have some of the qualities of the two elements which like to communicate warmly, Fire and Earth. And I think most of them are. Things get a little bit more complicated when I looked at more investigative journalists, those that are required, not so much to relate to us as to dig down and ferret out the news. And here, as I would expect, it is Water above all, with Metal following behind, which dominate. With Wood it appears to be those journalists often more directly involved in action.

I'm afraid that the list is of people perhaps familiar only to a British audience, particularly to those tuned to the BBC, but all can be viewed on YouTube or video extracts, if you are interested enough to track them down. I have also added names of other famous people, such as sports people and politicians, to plump out the list a little.

So here goes with my list:

Wood: Kate Adie, a former war correspondent, Caroline Wyatt (a current BBC defence correspondent), Peter Snow, Michael Gove

Fire: Evan Davies, Bruce Forsyth, Chris Evans

Earth: David Dimbleby, Fiona Bruce, David Attenborough, Jon Snow, David Cameron

Metal: Frank Gardner (a BBC defence correspondent). There must be more, but I haven't found anybody to add to the list yet.

Water: Robert Peston, John Humphrys, Jeremy Paxman, Gary Lineker, Arsène Wenger, Alex Ferguson, George Osborne, Ed Miliband

I find it interesting, and appropriate, that the Water element dominates the list, evidence of its ambition and desire to reach the top and stay there. Many of the heads of financial institutions who appear on TV regularly to defend the banks appear to be Water, too.

◇◇◇◇◇◇◇◇◇

18 FEBRUARY 2012
Don't let blocks block your mind

In a recent blog (8 January 2012) I wrote: 'Don't spend too long trying to diagnose the major blocks (Possession, Husband/Wife). They are much more difficult to diagnose than you may think. It doesn't matter if you miss them to start with. They become more and more obvious the longer they remain untreated. An expert practitioner may see them straightaway; a less experienced practitioner will inevitably take longer to recognize them. There is a risk that a newly qualified practitioner will over-diagnose blocks because of the excitement of doing them!'

Clearing Entry/Exit blocks and other blocks of all kinds forms an essential and highly effective part of five element practice. Detecting them is much more difficult than people think it is. There are two main reasons. Firstly, too many people think that it is only through the pulses that most blocks can be detected, and, secondly, and far more riskily, people assume that their pulse readings are accurate. The art of pulse diagnosis is so refined that even now, after nearly 30 years of taking pulses, I never rely only on my pulse readings to tell me if a block is there. It is always worth reminding ourselves that the 12 pulses our fingers are trying to interpret are an expression of the unique complexity, body and soul, of another human being. To interpret what they are telling us is therefore such a delicate, refined art, developed, with much humility, over many years of practice, that we should always add to what we think we are feeling other possible indicators of blocks to support our diagnosis.

Such indicators will consist of some physical or emotional evidence of blocked energy. For example, I may observe that a patient rubs their eyes or ears, or has some white mucus at the corner of their eyes, and, even before taking their pulses, I may already be thinking, 'Aha! II/III (SI/Bl) block!' Or they may complain of a bloated stomach or of sinusitis, and I think, 'Aha! X/XI (LI/St) block!' I may notice that the patient seems unexpectedly irritable today, and wonder whether the Wood element is blocked (VI/VII (TH/GB) block or VIII/IX (Liv/Lu) block). I may be surprised at a patient's colour, and see that it is whiter or redder than usual, and so on. All these are warning signs of some disturbance in the officials which I will add to my pulse diagnosis.

Finally, we were always taught that a Husband/Wife imbalance was life-threatening, because it shows stress on the Heart. If we do not diagnose this correctly to start with, don't worry, all you practitioners out there. No patient of mine has actually died because I failed to detect a H/W immediately. Obviously we need to clear it as soon as possible to relieve the pressure upon the Heart, but again I have never known a H/W block to be there without the patient showing quite obvious signs of deep distress to guide me to it.

◇◇◇◇◇◇◇◇

24 FEBRUARY 2012
Using our two hands

I have recently been thinking about the question of why some branches of acupuncture have taught their acupuncturists to use two hands to needle and to take pulses, and why others prefer just one. In five element acupuncture, or at least certainly how I was taught all those years back at JR Worsley's college in Leamington, we use both hands in both cases. Thinking about why this should be so, I decided to observe myself closely during my own practice to see how I felt about what I now do so automatically, and why I find great satisfaction in using both hands.

It isn't just because this is the way I was taught, although of course the comfort of an old habit is part of this. The main reason, I think, is because it feels good to me to enclose the needle in both hands as I guide it to the points. In doing this, I also maintain a comfortable contact with my patient's body. In taking pulses, too, both of my hands take my patient's hand and hold it against my body. I am using both hands to convey as sensitive and warm a touch as I can.

Pulse-taking and needling done in this way encompass something much more than just making physical contact to obtain some diagnostic information. It is possible to approach the skin with a needle without any of our fingers actually making contact with our patient's body, and pulses can be taken in a purely physical way, as we know from our visits to a doctor's surgery. Here there is no intention to convey anything through touch itself, which is so different from the importance five element acupuncture places on conveying warmth and comfort through our hands. As I observe the one-handed way of taking pulses or needling it always feels to me as if practitioners are holding the other hand well away from their patient as though to distance themselves from what they are doing.

Our hands can and should be able to convey protection, love or respect, still anger and calm fear, the five dominant emotions our treatments are trying to restore to balance. And they should continue to do this whenever we touch our patient's body, whether to take pulses or to needle or simply to make warm contact.

So each time I needle or take a pulse I am offering something which, though apparently purely physical in nature, becomes something much deeper if coming from my heart. Anybody hoping to make closer contact with the elements in their patients, and at the moment practising one-handed acupuncture, may consider taking their courage literally in both hands, and decide to learn to use both as a further expression of their care for their patients.

At a slightly different level, I shudder internally as I watch people needling a II/III (SI/Bl) block or a X/XI (LI/St) block on points around the eyes without tethering the patient's head with both hands, and making sure exactly where the eyeball is. What if the patient jolts their head, I think – and it can happen! And the reason I have heard practitioners give for not needling these points is precisely this fear. Using both hands reassures both patients and practitioners.

We are given two hands with which to embrace people, to cook with, to use a computer with, to drive a car with, why then do we cut ourselves so unnecessarily in half when we needle and take pulses?

◇◇◇◇◇◇◇◇

27 FEBRUARY 2012
A wise saying to make us think

I read this today in the *Guardian* newspaper:

'The radical Brazilian educator Paulo Freire once asked, "What can we do today so that tomorrow we can do what we are unable to do today?"'

This is such an acute question, and really made me think. Surely the purpose of each day should be to do something that makes tomorrow different and better.

◇◇◇◇◇◇◇◇◇

28 FEBRUARY 2012
David Hockney: a lovely example of the Fire element

I have just watched a warm interview with David Hockney, the painter, on BBC television, and smiled throughout. I wonder whether it is only a Fire person who could paint such delightfully joyous paintings of trees, with their ridiculous-seeming purple trunks and bright red branches. Somehow he even manages to make winter a joyous season.

Somewhat flippantly, this has made me wonder whether we can indeed diagnose artists through their artistic creations. I doubt, for example, whether a Metal person could see nature in the prime colours Hockney does, preferring instead, I would think, subtler autumnal shadings.

◇◇◇◇◇◇◇◇◇

3 MARCH 2012
The case for marking points before needling

I remember clearly being told by JR Worsley as a student that the most important reason for marking a point before needling is so that you know exactly where not to needle the next time when your first needle has not found the point. I always liked that. It made me more relaxed about my point location, because it somehow assumed that more than one needling would quite often be needed before we actually got the point. I also remember him telling us that it didn't matter how often we needled before we found a point. The important thing was to find it eventually rather than worrying how long it took us to find it. It is quite common for me to needle two or three times even now, and I don't find this at all odd. Instead, I am rather surprised when my needle accurately finds this infinitesimally small location first time.

If you are not sure where the AEPs (back shu points) are (and we all know how difficult backs can be), then, to be on the safe side when you are doing an AE drain, place needles down the Inner Bladder line not just where you think the yin AEPs are, but on points above and below these. In this way you cover all eventualities. It's far better to accept that locating points on the back is always difficult than to pretend that it's easy and miss the points for something as important as an AE drain.

Marking points is also important for another reason. It is good to get a view of the line of the meridian, rather than thinking of individual points in isolation. If you mark some part of the meridian line to help you orientate yourself, this provides you with a grid which can be seen when you stand back from the body. You will find that a wrong location often leaps out at you when seen from a distance in this way. For example, the three important upper Outer Bladder points, III 37–39 (42–44), can then be seen to be too low or too high, or it will become obvious that IV 24 (Ki 24) is marked at the wrong level, often too high on the chest in women, possibly because practitioners hesitate to ask their female patients to undo their bras to find this point.

Of course people reading this may say that we should not needle through points marked with a pen from a hygiene point of view (though does anybody actually know anyone of the many thousands of patients where points have become infected through doing this?). Nonetheless, good practice in the UK at least dictates that points should be marked with a small circle and the needle placed inside the circle. They can also be marked with a surgical pen, although these markings are difficult to remove and this should certainly not be done on the face.

We should always be prepared to use whatever aids we can to find points accurately and not be ashamed to do so. I certainly am not, and will continue to mark all points. I find it also concentrates my mind, as though the mere act of marking the point is already focusing my energy at that one spot.

◇◇◇◇◇◇◇◇

9 MARCH 2012
Preparing for my next trip to China

I am now preparing for my second visit to China at the end of this month where I will again be holding a two-week teaching seminar in Nanning. It is exciting to be going back so soon to see how far my students there have moved on in their five element studies, and to give further encouragement to their enthusiastic response to my first visit.

Through a dedicated website they have set up I have been sending them lessons at regular intervals which they are downloading with great diligence and in great numbers. I am therefore hopeful that I will find that they feel more confident about putting their newly acquired five element skills into practice in their own clinics.

On a happy note, too, I have been given an update on the sales of the Mandarin version of my *Handbook of Five Element Practice*. To my surprise and delight, the first print run was for 5000 copies of which 4500 have already been sold. The book is now being reprinted. It's lovely to think of 4500 people scattered around China all immersed in their five element studies!

◇◇◇◇◇◇◇◇◇

16 MARCH 2012
Let our patients surprise us!

It always pleases me to find how energized I feel after a day's clinical seminar, and the one just past is no exception. We had participants from Berlin, Dublin and the Netherlands as well as our usual core from England, something which, with my own half-European background, I really enjoy. And since quite a few had met each other before at other seminars I had given, there was the usual happy buzz of people catching up with one another.

The most important thing for me is the enthusiasm and receptiveness I can sense in the room, and the real keenness in all of us, me included, to learn more from the two patients participants had brought for diagnosis and treatment.

These seminars also provide a kind of a moving benchmark for me, as I realize that my years of practice have taught me more than I sometimes recognize. I can see that some of the signs of the elements I observe in patients are not as obvious to some of the class as they are to me. And this always reminds me of the many, many times I took patients to see JR, and he would say 'Fire' or 'Wood' or 'Water', and at first I simply could not see this, and only gradually came to realize that what at the time I thought in an over-simplistic way were the signatures of Fire or Wood or Water had to expand and change to accommodate what JR was teaching me.

Looking back I recognize, too, that this was really the only way to learn – through what I got wrong, not through what I got right, something he always told us, as our faces fell at yet another new and often initially puzzling insight into the mysteries of an element.

The words imprinted on our five element hearts should be, 'Humility, humility and yet more humility.' We should never be arrogant enough to think that we know all the deep secrets the elements hide within another human being. We should just be delighted, as I always am, that our learning is never finished, and that tomorrow's patient may open yet another new gate on to the landscape of the elements.

◇◇◇◇◇◇◇◇◇

24 APRIL 2012
Written before my return to London after my second visit to China

My second trip to China is now nearing its end and sitting here in the hotel room in Nanning, just gently thinking things through, I'm trying to summarize what I have taught my students and what the whole experience has taught me.

I have been listening to Mandarin spoken at full tilt and in great quantities by everybody around me, interspersed only with the pauses as the important parts were translated into English for me. I found it interesting to note that more and more of the few simple words I had learnt at my classes in London seemed to leap out of the sentences at me, like carp leaping out of the lake I visited here. And just for that moment the speech appeared to slow down as I recognized a word with some meaning I could attach to it, only for the remainder of the sentence to become submerged again in an unintelligible jumble of sounds. Although this was often confusing, as giving me only tiny glimpses of meaning, it was comforting to know that I had indeed started to learn something of the speech I heard around me. But what a long way to go before I can engage in any real dialogue here!

At a more serious level, I come away delighted that the students have learnt so much more than at my first visit, and that we have put together some solid structures for future learning. It is intended that I go over there twice a year, and Mei, who set in motion the whole train of five element acupuncture on its journey back to China, will probably go a further twice a year, as well as accompanying me. Her next visit is scheduled for July, so the students will get more time to consolidate what they have just learnt before I return with her in the autumn.

The number of my students has increased by a further five or so, making about 20 dedicated five element students. There are now two main groups, one based here in Nanning and the other in Chengdu, with a lone student hoisting the five element flag in Beijing. We will organize the website forum they have set up for me a little better, and they are arranging regular monthly meetings where they will help each other with their patients.

I call them my students, but they are all either fully practising acupuncturists or nearing qualification, so that their basic acupuncture knowledge is well established. If anything they have a much more solid foundation than comparable practitioners here in the UK, since they are blessed from birth with a deep understanding of the elements as forming an integral part of their life, so that we already speak the same language. This is so different from the UK, where I well remember one student, after about six months' training, asking, 'But how do we know that there really things like elements?' Here, by contrast, the elements represent the symbols through which life expresses itself.

By the last few days of this fortnight students had learnt some very fundamental components of five element practice, such as different needling and moxibustion techniques, how to carry out an AE drain, how to clear Possession and treat a Husband/Wife imbalance. Most important of all, I gave them a clear schedule of how to structure the first four treatments so that they feel confident that they know what to do at the start.

We saw together some 30 patients, and I treated at least another 25, because I gave each of the students a treatment. I felt it was important for them to experience an AE drain and their element source points for themselves, as many of them had not had any five element treatment before. Scheduling these treatments amidst the teaching sessions was a logistical puzzle which taxed my Small Intestine's ability to sort to its limit, but I managed the last three treatments on almost the last day. In doing this I only changed the element I had decided upon for one of the students, and I can only hope I am right with the others as I fly away to leave them to receive further treatment from their peers.

Each day was filled with treating patients, helping students treat patients, or helping them learn some of the five element skills they will need, such as testing for Akabane imbalance and learning how to apply moxa cones to salt for CV 8. This proved to be an unexpected very local problem, because the climate is so damp and they usually only use rock salt, that not only did the grains of salt stick together in a tight mass but the thick grains allowed the heat through too quickly so that I'm afraid I may have burnt the first person's umbilicus without realizing it. Being Chinese, she never complained of the pain and probably went away thinking that the pain was a necessary part of treatment. After this we found some thinner grains of salt, and worked out a way of putting rice grains in a little muslin bag to dry the salt out.

As usual, I learnt much from devising ways of teaching in such a limited and challenging timeframe.

◇◇◇◇◇◇◇◇◇

13 MAY 2012

A lesson in the spacing of treatments

I have been thinking a lot about the importance of the spacing of treatments after seeing two of my patients this week. We know that frequent, approximately weekly, treatments are essential at the start to allow a patient's elements gradually to regain strength and also to help us decide whether we are directing treatment at the right guardian element. So we don't have to think about the question of the spacing of treatment until more than about six treatments have been given.

Then, though, things start becoming a little more difficult, because we have to decide whether there has been sufficient improvement to make it sensible to space treatments a little more widely. I usually discuss this carefully with my patients and ask them whether they feel that they can manage a wider gap between treatments. I think this kind of discussion between us gives very useful feedback as to how patients really feel treatment is going, and gives them the opportunity to tell us if thing aren't progressing as they would like. We should never rely only on our own judgement of this, because many patients are reluctant to tell us how they really feel.

The important thing here is always to include patients in our deliberations about the spacing of treatment. Later on, when we have spread treatments even further apart, I will ask patients to tell me when they feel they would like to come back for their next treatment. And it is here that my two patients this week have taught me such a lot. Both are very long-standing patients, one having come for at least 15 years, the other for more than 20 years, and until quite recently I would leave it to them to contact me when they felt they needed a treatment. When I look at my notes, I realize that they both tended to do this at very infrequent intervals, one perhaps once or twice a year, the other often at longer intervals. And, then again from the notes, I notice that they would arrive very low in energy and needing at least a further two to three closely spaced treatments to get back on track. One of this week's patients, in particular, always left it far too long to get in touch with me, and would arrive very depressed and in need of a great deal of support.

About 18 months ago, I decided that I would look at things from a different angle, and instead of feeling that it would be inappropriate after so many years to suggest more frequent treatments, I would suggest that one of these patients would benefit from regular treatments every two to three months which we would arrange at each visit. This he accepted readily, particularly because, finances being a problem, I offered a reduced rate for each treatment, to suit his financial pocket at the time (he is a freelance actor). Once I had put this new regime in place, he immediately benefited from the more regular treatments, and told me this week that he was sure it was because of this that none of his physical symptoms had recurred and he had felt so well that he was able to accept more challenging work.

I then did the same with my second patient, and she, too, this week, told me how much this regular treatment had helped the changes in her life, which she ascribed, as did my first patient, to her frequent treatments. She now comes for a surprisingly brief booster every two months and feels her life has turned around since we have done this, mainly, I think, because the regular treatments have removed her feeling that she should be able to cope on her own.

Each patient's needs will be different. Some will clearly know exactly when they need a treatment, but in my experience such patients are rarer than those who are not sure themselves when they should phone us. Most of us will wait too long before we look for help, so I see it as the practitioner's task to decide with which patient to take a more active role in deciding when the next treatment should be and which patient we can leave to make the decision themselves.

I suspect that if I had introduced such a carefully graded plan for long-term treatment earlier on in my practice, I might have helped many more of my patients in the past. Looking back, there are many who I think would have benefited if I had been a bit firmer and clearer about the benefits of such a plan. So even at this late stage in my practice I find I learn new things.

I love writing about the wondrous effects simple five element treatments can have. This blog describes another example of this.

◇◇◇◇◇◇◇◇◇

22 MAY 2012
A good day in the clinic

There are times when I take what five element acupuncture can do a little bit too much for granted, but then I will find myself heartened by a treatment or series of treatments which reignites my wonder at what my needles have achieved. It also adds to my gratitude at having been given the chance quite late in my life (for I ventured into acupuncture in my mid-40s) to have found my way to a calling in which so much can be achieved with so very little – just through this comparatively tiny, one inch of flexible steel gently inserted to a comparatively very shallow depth in the skin, but able to stir the deepest depths within us all.

This has happened to me again this week, and fortunately, too, since I came back from China re-energized, only to fall foul of a bug of some kind which laid me low. I needed a good pick-me-up, and the one I am writing about today provided this so amply for me.

A new patient rang me in great distress. He had developed excruciating lower back pain, which was almost making it impossible for him to move. It sounded as if he needed what, in other disciplines, might be called emergency treatment. Here lies one of the traps for the unwary five element acupuncturist, because there is a myth deeply embedded in some acupuncturists' psyche that somehow five element acupuncture cannot treat acute physical conditions, and that five element acupuncturists need to look to other acupuncture disciplines to supplement what they do. This is something I have never understood, because it is belied by my many years of treating acute pain successfully using exactly the same treatment procedures as I use for any patient. And yet all of us, even the most experienced, when faced with an acute condition may feel an impulse to forget the carefully graded steps which start every course of treatment, and think first only of which points we could use in the area of the pain to counter it.

As we all know, these first steps consist first, and above all, of what we call a TD (a Traditional Diagnosis), followed by an AE drain and the source points of the element we have chosen. A TD should usually be as exhaustive as is necessary, firstly to set up a good relationship with our patient and then to find out as best as we may at this first encounter what is really going on in our patient's life. With acute pain, we may feel it better to shorten the bit of it we do face to face, only to continue it during the AE drain, an ideal time to do so for every patient. And in this patient's case, what I discovered was a great deal which helped explain why the backache was occurring just now, and was not just the first occurrence but a re-occurrence of one which had last occurred some 20 years earlier. This had been when his father had died and he had blamed himself ever since for not having reconciled himself with him before he died. Why did he think it might be recurring now, I asked him, and it turned out that his mother, too, had just died and all his feelings at this loss appeared to have brought to the surface the suppressed grief from long ago.

Reading this stated baldly like this, it might seem slightly fanciful to make these connections, but my patient certainly did not think so. And the strong reaction to his first treatment only confirmed this, because over the next few days he experienced feelings of deep grief, which made him examine his relationships to his own children, particularly his son. The most interesting thing from my point of view was that on his second visit a few days later he hardly mentioned his back pain, and when asked, said almost with surprise that, yes, it certainly seemed much better. By the third treatment the pain had completely disappeared, and he felt as he said, 'A completely new man.'

I hope this adds another nail to the coffin in which should lie buried the myth that five element acupuncture cannot treat acute physical symptoms.

For my acupuncture readers, I give below the very simple first three treatments I gave him, all, as you can see, directed at the Metal element.

Treatment 1: AE drain (a little AE on IX and V (Lu and HP))

X (LI) 4, IX (Lu) 9 (3Δ and needle)

II (SI) 19 – III (Bl) 1 (SI/Bl block – see next blog today for explanation)

X (LI) 4 – IX (Lu) 9 again (no moxa)

Treatment 2: CV 8 (3Δ on salt)

X (LI 20) – XI (St) 1 (LI/St block)

IX (Lu) 8, X (LI) 6 (3Δ and needle)

Treatment 3: III (Bl) 38 (42) (5Δ and needle)

X (LI) 11, IX (Lu) 9 (3Δ and needle)

◇◇◇◇◇◇◇◇

22 MAY 2012
Entry/Exit blocks, and when to do them

I have written before of the lure of the Entry/Exit block. I think this is because we all hope that we can achieve the often rapid easing of a painful condition that the clearing of such a block can do. But in fact we must not let our enthusiasm for this essential area of five element practice lead us to over-diagnose blocks.

In early treatment, as with the patient in my previous blog today, *A good day in the clinic*, I felt there was a II/III (SI/Bl) block immediately after the AE drain, but, as you can see, I did not clear it then, but needled the source points first. It was only after I felt the block was still there that I cleared it. As you can also see, I finished the treatment by returning to the source points, as we always should, but this time just doing a simple needling without doing moxa. You don't want to overdo things, particularly not at the first treatment.

The reason for waiting to gauge the effects of the source points is that we should try to address the element we are treating as soon as we can after the AE drain, and give it time to respond to this first treatment. Often the balance it tries to bring to the whole cycle of the elements reduces the pressure we can feel on the pulses which makes us think there is a block there. Even if we feel there is a Husband/Wife block after the AE drain, the same procedure holds true. We should needle the source points first, and then decide whether the pulse picture still indicates a H/W. Often the left–right discrepancy on the pulses disappears as the guardian element starts to take control.

So be careful not to put too much faith in your fingers' ability to diagnose blocks, and let the elements do as much work by themselves as they can. That does not, of course, mean that you should overlook blocks, simply wait a little to make sure that they are really there.

◇◇◇◇◇◇◇◇

31 MAY 2012
Spleen 4: a patient's comments

I love hearing how patients experience different points, so I give below something an Earth patient of mine said immediately after I needled XII (Sp) 4.

'Goodness, that's a lovely feeling. It feels as though there is a seeping of warm water all over my feet – like dense liquid.'

It is rare for patients to be so specific about the effect of treatment so soon after needling, although I always treasure in my own treatments the involuntary drawing up of my mouth and jaw into a smile as soon as my Small Intestine is needled, proof, if proof is needed, that Fire is to do with joy.

Modern life places different kinds of stresses upon different elements. Below I describe how my Earth element was affected by the deprivations of the war years.

Each element will be susceptible to its own kind of stress, none more so than the Earth element, which forms the centre of each our lives, and provides the stability which the shifting sands of modern life often undermine.

◇◇◇◇◇◇◇◇

7 JUNE 2012

Our relationship to food – and what it tells us about the element Earth

I have been thinking a lot about our relationship to food in a five element context. First, because I was asked by a fellow practitioner to help her treat an anorexic patient, and secondly, because I was made aware over this Jubilee weekend in London of my own often unbalanced relationship to the eating of chocolate.

Second things first: I have always attributed my odd cravings around chocolate to my upbringing during the Second World War when there was no chocolate in the shops. My family spent a major part of the war in what was then called rural Westmorland in flight from the Blitz in London. We rented a rat-infested little cottage by the lakeside in Bowness-on-Windermere, which had an old pre-war food kiosk in the road outside. In its window there was a display box of what were obviously paper chocolates, getting dustier by the day over the four years we were there. I would press my nose against the glass to look longingly at them, imagining to myself what they would taste like. Chocolates remained rationed long after the war ended, and being from a large family, we were each only allowed one small piece once a week. I always think that this may explain part of why chocolate is still something I yearn for, even though I can now buy as much as I like. Interestingly I hardly ever do, but if I am given a box, I will be hard put not to eat it all one go, as though making up for all those years of deprivation.

Buried in this personal story, though, there hides a great lesson about our understanding of the element which controls our attitude to food, the Earth element, our Mother element, and the element of hearth and home, which shelters the Stomach official and all that involves our relationship to food. And this brings me now to the anorexic patient. Food is inevitably associated with our mothers, and therefore with the kind of mothering, nurturing and feeding of body and soul which we each received as a child and which stamped itself upon how our Earth element deals with the food we are given. With eating problems of all kinds, whether those associated with over-eating or under-eating, we need to look at the kind of nurturing our patients received in childhood. If we look deeply enough, it will be there that we may find some explanation for what may later on have disturbed our patients' approach to food. In my own case, I feel it was no coincidence that, war child that I was, there were long periods when we were left in our grandmother's care to free our mother to return to London for weeks at a time to help our father with his London work.

It is revealing, too, to see the changes in body-shape which under- and over-eating cause. An anorexic person can appear to be shrinking gradually back down to their shape as a young child, as weight drops off, muscle loses its tone and menstruation ceases. An obese person moves in the opposite direction, as bulk is added. It is as though they are forming themselves into a shape which accommodates not only themselves but somebody else inside their skin. They appear to be enclosing themselves within something which could be said to offer the warm comfort of a home into whose arms they can sink. And this great envelope of flesh seems to be able to offer them an endless supply of food for a hunger that cannot be satisfied unless the deep underlying needs can be acknowledged and understood.

We may think that such imbalances in the Earth element point to this element being the guardian element in each of these cases, but that is not so. Any of the five elements, including Earth, may suffer from eating problems. The anorexic patient I saw this week was of the Wood element, and my element is Fire. In each case, though, it is our Earth element which takes on the burden (emotionally and physically) of whatever imbalance lies at the root of the problems.

Finally, since the actual level of food intake is the effect, not the cause, of a patient's imbalance, it is unhelpful to focus all our and our patients' attention upon the amount of food consumed, as many therapies dealing with eating problems do. Instead we need to help patients work out ways of dealing with the underlying problems, and this is done by strengthening the guardian element's ability to restore balance. My craving for chocolate, I always think, is more to do with my mother's absences from home and my fear that something might happen to her under the London bombings than to the rather sad paper chocolates in the kiosk window.

◇◇◇◇◇◇◇◇◇

17 JUNE 2012
The simpler the better

It is interesting how often I return to the phrase 'the simpler the better' when helping acupuncturists gain confidence in their five element skills. And I keep on repeating it because, much to my continuing surprise, what I say does not appear to be actually what people want to hear. It seems as if, instead, they prefer to believe the opposite to be true, that the more complicated things are the better they are.

One reason may be because people like to take pride in thinking that their discipline is a complex one requiring hard work to practise it. To encourage its practitioners to greater levels of simplicity may appear to run directly counter to this, as though it strips away some of this pride. It also takes courage to trust that minimum interference may mean maximum effectiveness, but there is no doubt in my mind that it does.

Nor must we think that it is easy to be simple, for this is far from the case. Some of the most sublime music ever composed is that of Mozart's piano concertos, where the pianist may only interject a single note as counterpoint to the orchestra. And yet if that note were placed a bar earlier or a bar later, or at a slightly higher or lower tone, the whole perfection of the musical structure would be broken. These single notes could appear to be written by a child, and yet they are the product of the highest level of creativity.

I like to feel that we can show some of this creative ability in our own work, if, instead of bombarding the elements with a plethora of points, often picked at random from one of those books on points I dislike so much, we dare to hone our selection down to a few simple points, and end on the single note of a command point. Treatment, like music, should then be allowed to fall silent, as we give the elements the time to carry on their healing work without further interference from us.

24 JUNE 2012

Walking in the street: a lesson in the elements

I have learnt something more about the Fire element and about myself this week. It seems that I need to interact with everybody I pass in the street, as though apparently trying to set up a fleeting relationship with those walking towards me. I can even find myself on the tip of talking to them (about the weather, or the state of the pavement, or whatever), and have to hold myself back. I am amazed at just how much effort I seem to be expending on these tiny, second-long interactions. What I am doing is trying to look in their eyes, if they will let me, in an attempt to evoke a response from them. And because I have been observing myself closely as I pass people, I am also observing them as they pass me. I have been passed by those who, like me, look me straight in the eye, by people who don't seem to notice I am there, but obviously must because they don't bump into me, by people completely absorbed in their own thoughts, by people careful to let me pass and by people simply brushing me aside.

Since Fire is the only element which needs to set up relationships wherever it finds itself, this has been the easiest element for me to carry out my mini-diagnoses on. The other elements are more difficult to detect in those few seconds of our encounter, but I have discovered all kinds of pointers in the way they notice or don't seem to notice me. So here are just a few rules-of-thumb (what an odd expression that is!*) when next you are out in the street:

---

* Just looked this up on Wikipedia: 'The term is thought to originate with wood workers who used the width of their thumbs (i.e., inches) rather than rulers for measuring things, cementing its modern use as an imprecise yet reliable and convenient standard.'

Fire looks into your eyes

Wood hurries to get past you

Earth is absorbed in their own thoughts

Metal looks through you

Water may glance at you but also all around you (as usual Water is the most difficult to pin down in this as in everything else it does)

Of course, all of us can do all these things, whatever our element, but these tiny pointers can be surprisingly useful in helping us understand the elements a little better.

Finally, none of the above holds true for those walking and talking on their mobile phones, in which case the Metal element will reveal itself in all of us whatever our element. We hold a metal object, the phone, and listen to words coming to us from the far-distant ether and send our own words back out there into distant space. No doubt in doing this we will all take on that Metal look of appearing to look through everybody we pass!

◇◇◇◇◇◇◇◇◇

26 JUNE 2012
A view from inside the Water element

I have just received some very illuminating insights into the Water element sent to me all the way from India by a friend of mine whose guardian element is Water. She wrote this after reading my blog on *Walking in the street* (24 June 2012).

'I read your recent blog, which was interesting. These short, simple observations of each element in a particular situation are very easy to remember and think about. It's also certainly a fact that on the street, I would look at people but immediately look away! I think it is because I don't want them to know that I am looking at them unless they want to initiate contact. If they smile, for example, I would spontaneously smile back and maintain contact for a short while before looking around. It's as if I feel I am transparent and everyone is always able to see through me (literally I mean) and that everyone is trying to read my mind and judge me. And I need to distract most people (except those I am very comfortable with) from something I may have been focussing on by looking here and there, away from what originally caught my attention. I think this is what partly causes the jerkiness that is experienced by others in Water. It's also as if I need to constantly check the environment to condition my own response or state of being to it, perhaps a bit like water which changes its state so often. This takes up a lot of physical and mental energy unconsciously in its own way (as Fire does in its attempt to reach out and every other element in their individual ways).'

◇◇◇◇◇◇◇◇◇

1 JULY 2012
Grief

I think the following is a beautiful description of the loneliness of grief, the feeling of isolation we all feel when we experience loss. It comes from a book by the American writer, Francine

Prose, called *Goldengrove*, which is all about how a young girl copes with the death of her sister.

'So many (of those trying to offer comfort) said the same things that I might have thought that there *was* common ground, if I hadn't known that I was alone on an iceberg split off from a glacier... When they wept, I cried, too, and for a moment I almost believed that my iceberg might have room for another person.'

◇◇◇◇◇◇◇◇

5 JULY 2012

Points are messengers, not the message

Some of you may have been surprised when I wrote in my blog of 17 June 2012, *The simpler the better*, last paragraph, that I dislike books which list the function of points. So here are my reasons.

We should always remember that points provide access to the meridians on which they lie, and through this to the elements deep within, each point a tiny opening through which external energies can be drawn in and down and internal energies drawn up and out. We sometimes forget this, because as acupuncturists we only work on the surface of the body, and our concept of the meridian network is often modelled too closely on the two-dimensional charts hanging on our walls. But though we use the points as places where we needle, their function is to convey the messages our needles are attempting to send down to the elements upon whose meridians they lie. They are therefore always messengers, never the message itself.

Books listing the various functions of individual points can confuse the unwary. If used carefully such books may well add to our understanding of the points, though I myself doubt much that is written in them, wondering upon how much actual clinical experience they are based as opposed to theoretical musings about the ancient Chinese meaning buried in their names. What worries me is that relying on these books for our point selection, which so many acupuncturists sadly tend to do, inevitably weakens the awareness of the link between point and element, and potentially makes a knowledge of the element secondary to the apparent function of a particular point. As five element acupuncturists, we are on a slippery slope once we begin to think of the point as having a function all its own quite distinct from that of the element which gives it that function.

We must never confuse the messenger with the message. And if our treatment is getting nowhere, we should not shoot the messenger (the points we have used), but look to change the message (the element on which they lie)!

<><><><><><><>

5 JULY 2012
The dark days are over!

Over the past years I have experienced many dark days when I despaired for the future of five element acupuncture. Now, I can say with heartfelt relief, no longer. It is not only that the whole of China appears to have opened up to welcome it back to its heart after many decades of absence, but in the UK, too, maybe perhaps partly as a result of this or because the spirit of the age demands it, five element acupuncture appears to have regained its soul. I see evidence of this all around me, and am deeply encouraged by it to continue my work in promoting it.

One small, but significant, evidence for this found its way round the world to me by a circuitous route, which illustrates how the world is now indeed one. Mei Long, my young Chinese student and friend, translates part of my blog into Mandarin for her own mini-blog (called a weibo), which then speeds on its way round China and to any Mandarin-speaker elsewhere in the world, where it apparently attaches itself in some form to Liu Lihong's blog, which is read by a vast readership in China. A reader of this blog is a young Chinese girl living in London who came to one of my seminars, decided to experience five element acupuncture for herself and now wants to study it.

Things do indeed come full circle if we wait long enough.

◇◇◇◇◇◇◇◇

16 JULY 2012
Dispelling a myth about moxa

It's lovely to get feedback from patients about successful treatments we have done. So here is something I can share with you.

A long-standing patient of mine told me that she had been suffering for some time from persistent menopausal hot flushes. Her element is Earth, and this is the treatment I gave her:

CV (RM) 12

III (Bl) 38 (or 43, if you prefer – which I don't!)

XI (St) 41, XII (Sp) 2

All the points were tonified and moxibustion was added to each point.

My patient was amazed by the effect of the treatment. The hot flushes stopped that night, and she hasn't experienced any since.

I hope this goes some way to dispel the widespread myth that moxa should never be used on patients suffering from hot flushes. The opposite is true. Whilst hot flushes make people feel very hot on the outside, they can remain very cold on the inside. Indeed I suspect that the inner cold may be the reason why the Three Heater is working overtime trying to provide heat, but in the wrong place. Moxa helps correct this imbalance by sending warmth deep within the body (and soul!) to the meridian network.

This is called treating fire with fire.

◇◇◇◇◇◇◇◇

3 AUGUST 2012

Social networking amongst cows

It isn't even April 1st, but a few days ago I heard on the BBC that a university somewhere is doing research into this very subject. Apparently cows are being fitted with some kind of device which will help researchers find out how much cows like to chew the cud together. They will monitor how far the milk yield goes up if cows are allowed to stay with their group, or down if they are separated from them.

I imagine the answer will be the obvious one, particularly to a five element acupuncturist. Presumably a happy cow will produce more milk than an unhappy cow, just as a happy person will lead a more productive life than an unhappy person.

◇◇◇◇◇◇◇◇

3 AUGUST 2012

Treating children with five element acupuncture

I love passing on heartening news about the results of simple five element treatments. And this latest anecdote, from the practice of a friend of mine, encouraged me to think a little more about our approach to treating children.

An 11-year-old girl suffering from severe migraine came for treatment. The practitioner felt that her element was Fire, and this is the first treatment she was given:

> AE drain: great deal of AE on IX, V and I (Lu, HP and Ht)
>
> Source points of Outer Fire: VI (TH) 4 and V (HP) 7

The migraines stopped completely the day after treatment, and have not recurred since. She will be given one more treatment in a few weeks' time (summer seasonal: VI (TH) 6: VI (TH) 6 and V (HP) 8), and will come back for occasional top-up treatment if necessary.

The migraines started after she moved school, leaving many of her close friends behind. She was also now being bullied by another child. All this meant that her Fire element was suddenly placed under a great deal of stress with which it could not cope. Hence the migraines and hence, too, the Aggressive Energy.

This made me think about the treatment I have given children, and why I have always, without exception, found Aggressive Energy to be there, and often a surprising amount of it for such young children. This then set me thinking about AE in general, and what its presence signifies. So why so much AE in children, when very sick adults may not have any?

I like to think that this may be because in children the imbalances are usually still at a fairly superficial stage, and have not had time to infiltrate deep within the elements. We were always told that AE was the result of one element under stress flinging the negative energy which is weakening it across the Ke (K'o) cycle to its grandchild element in an attempt to avoid harming its own child element. If the element under stress (which does not need to be the guardian element) has sufficient energy to get rid of negative energy in this way, it is still strong enough to maintain a good level of energy. An AE drain may therefore help to deal with the first attack on the elements, and it may be that it is only when elements are deeply weakened that more sustained treatment at a deeper level is required.

When we treat children, we use exactly the same five element protocols as for adults, but we use less of them and treat far less often. We don't need to treat children more frequently than once in two weeks, even at the start of treatment, and then only for a few treatments, spreading treatments out more quickly than for adults. We also use less moxa on the points (though children will be fascinated by moxa if you show a cone being heated on yourself first to calm them). We also needle on one side of the body only, to reduce the stress for a child, except in the case of the AE drain and Entry/Exit blocks.

We also have to get used to needling a struggling child! I use short needles, and always hold the needles carefully covered by my hand so that the child doesn't see them. It is important to needle quickly, and not delay things by trying to talk a child through its fear, as you would with an adult. With the AE drain, if the child is young enough I ask the parent to take the child on their lap, and hold the child very firmly as I insert the needles. The needles often fall out when the child struggles, so have a good supply to hand.

And pulse-taking in these circumstances is also quite difficult! So we do our best with whatever information we have. Obviously, too, we have to learn about the child not only by observing it ourselves for as long as we can, but by talking to the parent(s)/guardian. Again, obviously, this should if possible be done when the child is not present. A phone call or meeting before the first treatment, in which we ask the parent/guardian the kind of questions we would ask an adult at the TD (Traditional Diagnosis), is essential to give us a picture of what is going on with the child and the family's approach to this.

What is interesting, though, is that children themselves respond very quickly to the effects of treatment. Though they may shriek or struggle a bit, the little child who makes a terrible fuss about the actual needling will often be the one who rushes into the practice room and greets me with a kiss, as though it knows I have helped it.

The important thing is always to bear in mind that the reason why a child needs treatment is, as we know, not simply because of something physical, but, as with any patient we treat, inevitably has a deeper emotional cause. All those terrible cortisone inhalers now lined up on primary school shelves which the young children are told to take for their asthmas could be thrown away if only people realized the stress their children's Metal elements are placed under in this modern world. When we are asked to treat children, therefore, we must always look beyond the child first to the parent(s), and then beyond the parent to the world in which the child lives.

Usually, unfortunately, we are not asked to treat the parent, although we can clearly see that this is where the trouble lies. In the case of this young girl, it seems that her parents may not appreciate how much the change of school and the bullying is affecting their child, and in this way are not acting to support the child's Heart Protector in a way that will help it protect itself from the bullying. As we know, bullies always pick on a child which shows weakness, so the stronger its Heart Protector becomes, the more it will be able to stand up for itself.

◇◇◇◇◇◇◇◇

6 AUGUST 2012
Usain Bolt: Fire!

You can't have a better example of Fire than Usain Bolt. Anybody who can make a whole stadium of people smile, let alone the billions watching on TV, must be Fire. And he loves acting the clown.

Apart from enjoying the Olympics, which have lit up the UK with a very English kind of enjoyment, I love watching how the different athletes respond to the stresses and joys of competition from a five element point of view. It's fascinating seeing all the different expressions of the elements so clearly visible, and there's no better way of adding to our knowledge of the elements than watching people under stress.

◇◇◇◇◇◇◇◇◇

11 AUGUST 2012
Usain Bolt Part 2: A further lesson on the Fire element from the Olympics

I have been watching Usain Bolt very carefully, trying to work out whether he is Outer or Inner Fire. I think now that he is Inner Fire, or, as we five element acupuncturists say, a II CF, with the Small Intestine as his dominant official.

Watching him has made me look again at the differences between these two sides of Fire. And there are great differences. I remember saying to JR Worsley that I thought there were really six CFs (guardian elements), not just five, because Fire could be considered to consist of two, and he nodded.

So here is what my observation of Usain Bolt tells me about what I see as being typical of the Small Intestine:

He is able to multi-task in a way very familiar to me from my own Inner Fire abilities, and in a way no Outer Fire person would do. I realized this when I saw him chatting happily to one of the stadium volunteers standing behind him just before the 200 metre final only a minute before settling down in his blocks. He is obviously able to switch quickly from one task to the next without apparently any loss of focus. This may even be his way of concentrating more on the next thing, even if this is an Olympics final.

He likes to include everybody in his joy, chatting to all his fellow competitors after the race, talking into the camera, running up to the crowd and talking to everybody there. Remember that the Small Intestine is the closest official to the Heart, and it wants to help the Heart express joy, particularly at these very intense moments. Contrast this with Jessica Ennis drawing her joy back into herself when she won, and her quiet self-absorption throughout the heptathlon. (I think she is probably Metal, so quiet and self-contained.)

He has great awareness of what is going on all around him, seeing exactly which camera is on him, responding quickly with a joke and a smile when he knows the world is looking at him. He watches everybody and everything all the time, as though using his Small Intestine's ability to sort so that it can send the right information on to the Heart.

◇◇◇◇◇◇◇◇

3 SEPTEMBER 2012
Hidden delights of London: Phantom Railings

If you walk from Gower Street to the back of the British Museum, at the corner where Keppel Street meets Malet Street, you will find the most delightful sound installation called 'Phantom Railings: an interactive sound sculpture'. The old iron railings along a high wall surrounding the gardens at the back of Gower Street were removed during the Second World War to be used for the war effort, as all railings were, and for some reason have not been replaced. You can still see the metal stumps left behind. As I walked past, my walk was interrupted by loud plinking and plonking noises. I stopped and looked around to see where they were coming from, only for the noises to stop, too. When I started walking again, the noises started up again, and I realized they were being controlled by the pace of my steps. By this time I had reached the large gates to the garden, which displayed a notice explaining that this was an installation 'to evoke the phantom of a lost iron fence'. The footsteps of passers-by recreate the sound of somebody running a stick along metal railings.

Delighted with this unexpected source of art displayed so discreetly in quite a hidden corner of Malet Street, I walked up and down several times, changing the speed of my steps and creating my own tiny symphony of sound.

And to round off my morning, I settled down to an Espresso at a little café round the corner, only to be charged £1.00 for it, the cheapest in London yet right in the centre of town. And it was served with a smile and piping hot, just as I like it!

What pleasures we come across in such unexpected places!

<><><><><><><>

25 SEPTEMBER 2012
Thoughts on another difficult practice situation

Please note that the title of this blog does not say 'how to deal with a difficult patient'. It is not that patients are simply difficult in themselves, but that we as people find them difficult to deal with. For practitioners, that is a crucial difference. As Shakespeare might have said, 'the fault lies not in our stars (or in this case our patients) but in ourselves…'

So here goes about this particular difficult situation. The patient was one who came for treatment as part of a clinical day I spent helping another practitioner with his patients. She is a woman of 35 and moves around in a wheelchair. Her medical notes show that she was diagnosed as autistic and with attention deficit problems as a child. She has a long list of other medical conditions, the main being a spinal accident which left her confined to bed for a year when she was eight and meningitis when she was ten.

What interested me was noting that she appeared to be quite capable of moving without help from the wheelchair to the treatment couch, nor did she have any difficulty in turning over on the couch. Her legs, too, did not have the look of ones where the muscles have atrophied from little use. She was wearing very heavy short boots, much like men's army boots, which looked incongruous on a wheelchair-bound person by reason of their sheer weight alone. She brought with her a little doll, the kind a five-year-old child might have, which she insisted on tucking next to her on the couch. I also noticed other disconcertingly odd things which made me question how far she was actually incapacitated.

Having expected from the notes that contact with her might be difficult because of her autism, I was surprised to see how easily she seemed to relate to us, and in particular noticed that she was darting hidden glances at me when she thought I wasn't watching.

The practitioner is also her medical practitioner, and had started his five element treatment by relying only on her medical diagnosis rather on a much more extensive five element diagnosis which would not have concentrated so exclusively on her physical conditions. The distinction between his role as her physician and as her acupuncturist had become understandably blurred. Initially, I, too, made the mistake of going along with this.

The practitioner and I therefore assumed all sorts of things about her condition, basing ourselves on very little information about her current medical condition. Did she in fact need a wheelchair at all, and could she be described as still being 'autistic'?

As is obvious to any five element acupuncturist from what I have written, we decided to treat her with Internal Dragons. We followed this with an Aggressive Energy drain and the source points of her element, which I thought was Fire. I had a question mark around Inner Fire (Small Intestine), something to do with the quickness of her understanding (even though she didn't like to show that she did understand) and the sharpness of her glance!

I felt surprisingly angry at the end of the treatment, as though she had got under my skin and had outmanoeuvred us. And I went so far as to tell the practitioner that I wasn't sure there was any point in continuing treating her with acupuncture because she appeared to be manipulating the situation in a way that made treatment impossible.

It was my anger which brought me to my senses, and I told the practitioner later that I did not think I had dealt properly with the situation. I had failed to take the right steps to get her treatment back in the correct five element groove. We should have done a proper Traditional Diagnosis after the treatment in whatever time we had available, to be continued at the next treatment. She should be asked to demonstrate how far she can stand and walk by herself, and the practitioner should get some answers to more detailed questions about her life. We were not even clear about her living situation. Does she live alone or with her family? Does she have friends? What does she do with her time?

But all is not lost. I have suggested to the practitioner that he should now start as though from scratch, trying to forget the wheelchair and the label of autism. Nor must he allow himself to be manipulated back into the old relationship where she appeared to be dictating how she wanted him to treat her. My mistake was to allow her to do the same to me.

This is the only way in which we can help this patient. And we should try to do that, rather than walk away. She is really crying out for help, and has probably been crying out for this help all her life in the only way she knows how.

It may be helpful to read this blog in conjunction with my blogs of 13 September 2011, *Losing control in the practice room*, and of 9 October 2011, *Regaining control in the practice room*, which complement this blog and deal with other problems in the practice room.

And so my learning continues.

◇◇◇◇◇◇◇◇

23 SEPTEMBER 2012
The pluses and minuses of life

It's funny how often I come across some quotation which seems particularly relevant. A few days ago, I read the following in, of all things, a detective story: 'Things always have to even themselves out between plus and minus. Between going forward and going back. That's the only way to live.'

I like to think that life has to balance itself between pluses and minuses (acupuncturists would say, between yin and yang). We tend to hope, unrealistically, that somehow the life we live should always be lived on the plus side. Far better to accept that every plus needs its minus. This brings the necessary tension which moves us towards change. Time always hustles us along despite ourselves, jolting us out of complacency, as a minus does its companion plus and plus its minus, and as yin its yang and yang its yin.

Interesting to find such a potentially deep thought tucked away between the covers of a simple detective story.

As I read though my blogs to see how many of them warrant inclusion in this book, I see how often I write about how my own understanding of the different elements gradually deepens the more I practise and observe. Whereas my thoughts in the books I have written remain as though fixed for ever in time, which is the time at which I wrote them down, these much smaller snippets of thoughts in this blog are added to or amended as time passes, so that a reader is able to see these thoughts in process of development. I, too, re-reading my blogs carefully, as I am doing now, am surprised to see how much I have used the medium of my blogs as a way of encouraging my ideas in this development. I now see for the first time how different this process is from the final end-result represented by writing a book, obviously the same process some of my readers go through as they make their way from blog to blog.

◇◇◇◇◇◇◇◇◇

30 SEPTEMBER 2012
My relationship to Metal – another new insight

I learnt something new about my relationship to the Metal element this week as a result of treating one of my Metal patients. At one point during the treatment I found that I was talking too much, and noticed that my patient only seemed to talk after prompting from me. The two-way communication I was engaged in appeared to be heavily weighted towards one side, where I was doing the talking, whilst the other side, my patient, was mostly doing the listening.

This set me wondering afterwards how far this was in general true of my interaction with Metal, and I decided that it was. I then looked at my interactions with all Metal people, and found that as a general rule it is as though Metal needs to wait to hear what I have to say before entering the conversation. I interpret this as a sign that Metal wants to assess the quality of what I am saying before deciding whether and how to take part in a dialogue with me.

I have now gone on to look at where my interactions with Metal might differ from those with patients of the other elements. The most obvious difference here is in the case of Fire, because, unlike Metal, it is generally unhappy with the kind of silence Metal feels at home with. A Fire patient is likely to be the one to start talking even as they come into the practice room, although, being a Fire practitioner myself, the chances are that they will have to be very quick of tongue to outpace my own need to speak to them!

Earth, too, is one of the elements most consistently engaged in speech, a sign of its need to make the listener understand what is going on for them. Conversations with Earth patients may sometimes be more in the nature of a monologue than a dialogue unless the practitioner steers the talk carefully. Wood may also need no prompting to talk if it has something it needs to say, and wants to make sure the practitioner is listening to what they are being told. Again, here, speech can descend into a monologue if the practitioner loses control.

Finally, my verbal interactions with Water patients always seem to have a very distinctive character of their own, which makes of them not so much a dialogue where one person talks, then listens whilst the other person talks, but a conversation where both talk at the same time in a kind of concerted murmur. It is as though the sound of the words, rather than the meaning of the words, is more important, offering the kind of reassurance that Water is not alone, which it craves in order to still its fear.

Of course, all these observations are based on the fact that my own reaction to everybody I come into contact with will be strongly coloured by my own Fire element. In trying to look at their own experiences with patients, each practitioner must therefore take into account how far their own guardian element shapes the way they interact with their patients and their patients interact with them.

I am now determined to watch myself more closely to see whether my own talking in the practice room is an appropriate response to the needs of my patient rather than an inappropriate response to my own needs.

◇◇◇◇◇◇◇◇

6 OCTOBER 2012

Insights into a Water person's relationship to the elements

I have just received the following comments all the way from India from a young Indian friend of mine written after she had read my blog of 30 September 2012, *My relationship to Metal – another new insight.* Her guardian element is Water. She is not an acupuncturist, but has been treated with five element acupuncture and as a result has developed a great interest in our approach.

'I read your last blog with great interest as I could almost visualize the nature of the conversations.

Conversations are one important way I try and look for elements as I am not often able to sense the colours or smell or sound (sometimes I can). More than the exact words, I often focus on how the conversation proceeds, how the other person talks and what I feel.

I don't think a lot of what you have described rests upon your needs or temperament in the clinic (except perhaps how you might judge the net result of a conversation) because I have very similar feelings while dealing with the elements, coloured of course by my own element.

What I mean is: Initially I always had a difficult time with Metal because it was hard to sustain a conversation. I always felt they were judging me and I was not holding their interest sufficiently. I also tend to talk more under these circumstances (sometimes I clam up, but that depends on whether I am trying to reach out or whether I don't want to have anything to do with the person). However, I suppose my kind of talk in this case would be different from a Fire person's. I just talk about whatever I can manage to think up every moment; it is sometimes fruitful and informative (as Metal people carry a lot of information with them) but not a relaxed kind of conversation.

I also have a problem with Earth because of the tendency of Earth people to direct the conversation so strongly and to easily (and illogically) overrule things that I might mutter or mumble (and I would only say those things once before retreating and letting Earth take its course). Earth is such a strong element in its manifestation – I feel they have a strong maternal aspect radiating from them but this is not something that draws me to them or that warms me. It is based somehow more on their needs rather than on being sensitive to mine, though they may be well intentioned.

Fire is the element I am most comfortable with. I am not always relaxed in their presence but I don't need to worry about taking charge of conversation and I know that many Fire people will actually want to listen to what I say. Even though they are doing a lot of talking, they are good listeners.

Wood is hard again and even when Wood is not pushy, there is always a latent tension inside me hoping that the push will not come suddenly and unexpectedly.

Water – I find it hard to recognize many Water people! I do recognize some and in those instances, even if external appearances of the element are different from mine, I can understand their behaviour. I find (especially lately) my voice certainly has a droning tendency and I do sometimes interrupt people in the middle of what they are saying (and I am trying not to do this because people naturally do not like this!) I think it is sometimes because I am afraid that I will not be able to express myself on some matter (i.e. the conversation may drift to something else or people may not hear me) and sometimes the desire to share something is so strong that I impulsively chime in. I think these are two different (positive and negative or yin and yang or however one may describe them) aspects of Water that motivate me to react in a seemingly similar way but with different reasons, during conversations.'

It is very rewarding for me to see how an understanding of the elements can help a person in their interactions with other people in their daily life. Thank you, Sujata, for your insights.

◇◇◇◇◇◇◇◇◇

1 NOVEMBER 2012
Whole-family treatment

I often say to patients who come with apparently intractable family problems that it is not selfish for them to concentrate on getting themselves into balance, because the changes in them will inevitably have a ripple-on effect on all the people around them. Often I see quite amazing improvements in the dynamics of a family as a result of the treatment of one of its members.

I witnessed one such change this week, when a patient, who had spent the past 20 or so years of her life trying to cope with the trying demands of her close-knit family, told me that over the past six months things had changed to such an extent that the entangled relationships which had so far made her feel so trapped were slowly resolving themselves. She is now strong enough to demand that instead of bowing to her family's needs they must now take her needs into account. As a result, there has been a change in all her relationships to her parents and siblings; with some she now feels much closer, with others she has learnt to keep her distance. And their relationships with each other also appear to have changed for the better.

In effect, we could say that our work makes us into family therapists.

◇◇◇◇◇◇◇◇

4 DECEMBER 2012
Back from China!

I return from China, humbled. We take so much for granted in our five element acupuncture in the West. The word 'spirit' is so deeply entrenched in our thinking that we can hardly visualize our work without this deep aspect of ourselves imbuing all that we do. This is so far from the modern Chinese view of acupuncture that it has taken me my three visits to understand the breath of change which I bring with me. Now, though, it is quite clear to me that what China's traditional medicine so desperately needs is to regain its spiritual roots, something so sadly suppressed over the past 30 years or more. And the prime mover in all this is my host, Liu Lihong. It is for this that they feel that what I have to offer is so badly needed over there.

So I taught and I talked for three weeks. We supervised the treatment of over 60 patients (this time mainly given by the acupuncturists who had come to our previous seminars rather than by Mei and me). I then gave two large seminars, one to 250 students at a traditional medicine college in Nanning and another to a large conference in Chengdu in a hall packed with 300 people with another 200 or so watching by video link. The difference in atmosphere compared with last year's conference was quite marked. Then I was talking as a rather lone voice, not exactly in the wilderness, but certainly to an audience many of whom were unfamiliar with any concept of five element acupuncture. This year, I felt as though I was amongst friends all eager to learn more.

And so many do! All are asking where they can learn. And there are so few of us to do the teaching! This is a challenge indeed, both for my Chinese hosts, who have difficulty in restricting the numbers to a reasonable amount, even to fit into the rooms available, and a great challenge for me, too. The only way we can see to meet such a demand will be to for me to devise some form of distance-learning based upon the Mandarin version of my *Handbook*, which was again handed out to everybody in their conference packs. We will also need to encourage the kind of self-instruction or working together in small groups which the original pioneers of acupuncture in the UK in the 1950s had as their only source of tuition. I told them that JR and his group of fellow explorers had to make do with only the few spare weeks of instruction a year then available to nourish their curiosity, and had to go off afterwards and explore for themselves what they had learnt. The rest of their learning was up to their own experimentation and determination. This is, after all, how JR came to develop his own insights into the role of the CF, Dick van Buren his theories about stems and branches and Mary Austin to devise her own five element approach. I encouraged everybody to be brave enough to act as pioneers for five element acupuncture's return to China.

Luckily for us they start from so much higher a level of understanding of the concept of the elements than any Western person has to begin with, for the elements are bred into them, as real to them as their life's blood, and they can quote verbatim and from memory from the *Nei Jing*. The majority of those coming to the seminars are practising, well-qualified acupuncturists, trained to a much higher technical standard, I felt, than many practitioners over here (no need to remind any of them of point positions or point names). They were therefore much, much quicker at making the slight adaptations to their techniques, such as pulse-taking or needling, demanded by changing to a five element approach.

Plans are well in hand already for my return in April, this time accompanied by both Mei Long and Guy Caplan. The student group will now expand from the 50 we taught this time to a further 50, making 100 students in all. Of these some of the original group will be ready to start teaching the new learners what they have learnt. And so the circle widens.

Now I need to get over my jet lag and start working on a more schematized distance-learning approach which will eventually be available for downloading by those in China. Quite a stimulating project to come back to!

◇◇◇◇◇◇◇◇

13 DECEMBER 2012

Five element thought for the day – some pointers I use to help trace an element's signature

Last week I had a very heartening day up at the Acupuncture Academy, the new college in Leamington, getting my first glimpse of a new group of students there, all eager to learn.

One of the things I told them was not to worry about feeling that there is any quick way to develop the complex skills required to distinguish those much-emphasized sensory signs the elements imprint on all of us. When I first started my studies, I think I was very optimistic about how easily I would perceive these, imagining that by the end of our three-year course I would be well on the way to assessing accurately all the four aspects of colour, sound, smell and emotion.

I was to find that this was far from the case, so far, indeed, that it was only after quite a few years of practice that I at long last began to understand what a rancid smell was, or honed my assessment of Earth's colour, yellow. And just when I thought I had 'got' one manifestation, I would find all my previous learning confounded by discovering that my patient's rather bright red face was nothing at all to do with Fire, but was either Wood or Earth out of balance. In the case of Wood, I eventually worked out that it was its imbalance which was throwing its child, Fire, out of balance and creating the red colour, and in the case of Earth, the red was coming from problems handed down to it by its mother. Fire, I have found, never imprints a constant high red colour on those of its element. Its reddish tinges come and go, as it flickers, but they never remain a constant imprint.

Now that I have recognized for myself how difficult it is accurately to perceive the elements' sensory signals, I realize how important it is for those new to five element acupuncture not to rely too heavily on sensory impressions which may well be leading them astray. Instead, I try to emphasize all the many other ways the elements reveal themselves, and share with them the observations I have accumulated over the years to help fill out what I lack in sensory awareness. For example, I have now developed for myself a list of the small variations in facial expression which help me pinpoint an element more clearly. I give these below as an aide for others.

Wood: Look at the eyes (perhaps obviously enough since Wood is to do with vision in every sense). Its eyes have a direct, often challenging look as though demanding a response from me. A secondary point may also be very tight neck muscles around the mouth or neck.

Fire: Look for the smile lines around the eyes. All elements smile when they are happy, or want to pretend they are happy, but only in Fire do the smile lines around the eyes stay in place long after the smile has faded. I can feel this in myself. I love warming my own Heart up by smiling, often doing this when I am on my own as my own personal comfort blanket. I now recognize Fire by those smile lines indicating that a smile is trying to force its way through.

Earth: The mouth: often slightly open, or if not open, then looking as if it would like to open, as though appealing for food.

Metal: The eyes, like Wood, but with a completely different look. They are not trying to set up any relationship with me, as Wood's eyes try to do, but even when looking at me seem to be looking past me as though into the far distance.

Water: Again the eyes, but here it is the movement of the eyes which is revealing. They have nothing like the stillness of Metal's eyes or the forcefulness behind Wood's gaze. Instead they seem to flicker, dart around, as though constantly on the move, ready to perceive danger and avoid it.

If all else fails, and you are not at all sure which element your patient is, then see whether the rather basic signposts I have listed above help you. I have found them to be a remarkably accurate way of supplementing what my senses are unable to tell me. And as you move on in your practice, you will also find your own pointers to add to this list – maybe a characteristic way of walking, or talking, holding a hand out for pulses to be taken or settling on the treatment couch. Since everything we do is the work of the elements within us, every part of body and soul will be showing characteristic pointers to our guardian element. We just need to be patient enough and give ourselves the time needed to develop our own individual stock of diagnostic pointers.

I still find it fascinating that each patient I see teaches me just a little more about the elements, and this learning will never stop since we are all unique manifestations of the interplay of the elements within us.

◇◇◇◇◇◇◇◇◇

19 DECEMBER 2012
My delight in a simple treatment

I always like to write about the satisfaction of doing what I do, and here is another confirmation of how effective a simple treatment can be. A few needles and a transformation.

I was called to the bedside of a very old friend of mine who I had treated many years ago. She had recently lost her partner of 50 years, and then had immediately to have surgery on both eyes for a glaucoma-induced condition. And now she had been diagnosed with severe atrial fibrillation. The eye surgery had left her with very blurry sight, and she was too giddy to walk by herself.

On the train to see her, I mulled over what treatment I thought I would need to give. The lovely thing about being a five element practitioner is that we have the pillars of five element treatment to call upon whatever the conditions we are faced with. I already knew her element was Wood. There had been no evidence of Possession when I talked to her at her husband's funeral, so that left only the AE drain, the possibility of a Husband/Wife imbalance and Entry/Exit blocks to consider. There proved to be very little AE, just a touch on Heart Protector and Heart, drained in just a few minutes. But a Husband/Wife imbalance was calling out loudly to me, both in her look of quiet, passive desperation, and in her pulses, which, though low on both sides, felt appreciably stronger on the right side.

There was an immediate change in her once I had cleared the H/W; her colour became less drawn and she said that her palpitations had died down. She lay back, closed her eyes and looked more at peace. I searched for other blocks, and found a II/III (SI/Ht) block. For good measure, I also did a VI/VII (HP/GB) block, even though it was not clear from the pulses. But the history of trauma surrounding her eye surgery made me think that I should do this, particularly as I never rely solely on my pulse readings to diagnose blocks.

I then needed to do something to strengthen her spirit so that the H/W did not recur, which was possible in view of all that she had to deal with. I had to decide between IV (Ki) 24 (a resuscitation point for the spirit after great trauma) or CV (RM) 14 (with its direct effect upon the Heart), and opted for CV 14 to help her Heart. I finished the treatment with the source points of Wood. I used no moxa for any of the points, because she has slightly raised BP. As I left her to sleep, she said, 'I feel a lot better, Nora.'

The next day she phoned me to say that she felt completely different, much more optimistic and less despairing. Her eyesight was clearer, she no longer had palpitations, she had climbed the stairs without becoming breathless, and was steady enough on her feet to go for her first walk unaided.

Here again is the list of points I used:

AE drain

H/W

CV (RM) 14

II/III (SI/Bl) block

VI/VII (TH/GB) block

VII (GB) 40, VIII (Liv) 3

All in all I could not ask for more from one treatment. How I love doing what I do!

◇◇◇◇◇◇◇◇◇

31 DECEMBER 2012

Some thoughts on the history of traditional Chinese medicine in China over the past 50 years or more

To understand the history of traditional Chinese medicine in its modern context better, I have been fortunate to have had recommended to me by a student at the Leamington Acupuncture Academy an excellent book which I have just finished reading with great interest, *Chinese Medicine in Early Communist China, 1945–63: A Medicine of Revolution* by Kim Taylor (Routledge, 2005). This is providing me with great insights into why my advent in China seems to be marking quite a turning-point in China's own appreciation of its traditional medicine, specifically in relation to acupuncture. It is certainly helping me understand a little better why what I bring represents a reconnection to an acupuncture tradition in great danger of being lost.

I would recommend all acupuncturists to read this book. It confirms many of my long-held beliefs about the problems surrounding modern Chinese acupuncture, known, somewhat confusingly, as TCM (traditional Chinese medicine), and its insidious spread into the West under the illusion that it somehow represents traditional acupuncture, which it so clearly doesn't. Thank goodness that this is at last being recognized, not least in China. But TCM's invasion of the West has done much untold harm to the more traditionally based practices of acupuncture in the UK, such as five element acupuncture, one such instance being the fact that, for some reason I could never fathom, TCM practitioners always seem to want to undermine the validity of five element acupuncture. Now, at least, I feel my own stance, staunchly defending the transmission of a long acupuncture lineage, has been vindicated by what is now being revealed about the extreme paucity of any true traditional sources in the acupuncture practised over the past 50 years or more in modern China.

My thoughts have been further strengthened by reading another important and well-researched book by Volker Scheid, *Currents of Tradition in Chinese Medicine, 1626–2006* (Eastland Press, 2007). Although concentrating almost entirely upon herbal acupuncture, with only a handful of references to acupuncture, the picture he paints is of the enormous pressures placed upon Chinese medicine over the past 50 years or more in what can be seen as a fight for its survival against the forces within China supporting the primacy of Western medicine. Chinese medicine became a pawn in China's attempts to work out the position it should take in relation to Western medicine, and continues to suffer from this uncertainty, whilst at the same trying to defend the importance of acknowledging its own long medical heritage.

Somehow acupuncture found its own escape route from the political turmoil within China, benefiting from the hounding and expulsion of many of its practitioners. They took with them, often as the sole inheritors of long traditional medicine lineages, traditional practices frowned upon or misunderstood in mainland China, and were free in the West to pass on their knowledge to those eager to learn. Amongst these, as we know, were the group in England which included JR Worsley and Dick van Buren.

Ironically, therefore, it is in the West that the precepts of traditional acupuncture found fertile ground upon which to allow its damaged roots to re-plant themselves and grow so prolifically. It is therefore doubly ironic that it should fall to me, a Western-trained five element acupuncturist, to hand the gifts which my practice has given me back to a birthplace which hardly recognizes the acupuncture inheritance on which I base this practice.

This is an important blog with which to round off my third year of blogging. I think it describes accurately and succinctly why I regard my mission to reintroduce five element acupuncture to China as so important.

2013 BLOGS

It is appropriate that I should start the new year 2013 with a blog about my new venture, the writing of my Teach Yourself Manual for the revised edition of my *Handbook of Five Element Practice*. I have now completed this, and it will be published by my new publishers, Singing Dragon, during the year. That formed the principal task for last year, slotted in amongst other projects of mine, such as travel to both China and various European countries to continue my postgraduate teaching.

This year has also been punctuated by the bout of ill-health I suffered during the summer, which prevented me from undertaking either of the two planned further journeys to China and some European visits. So this has proved quite a challenging year in many ways, which has forced me to re-assess what I am doing, how much I am doing, and look at whether I am working too hard or whether I can continue as before, now that I feel fully recovered.

2013 BLOGS

◇◇◇◇◇◇◇◇

5 JANUARY 2013
Five element distance-learning course

I am very much enjoying working on a distance-learning course for my Chinese students. It is quite an intellectually demanding challenge to shape the course, and decide what to include and what to omit. Luckily I have my *Handbook of Five Element Practice* to base it on. I wrote this some years ago, rather quickly, to help my SOFEA students, and on re-reading it now, I'm glad that it will provide a good foundation for those in China wanting to expand their acupuncture skills to include five element acupuncture.

I have completed ten lessons so far, with suggestions on practical work to accompany selected studies of the text. I will expand this to about 16–18 lessons so that by the end of the course I hope that those who are already acupuncturists will feel sufficiently confident to start practising five element acupuncture, and those who are just interested lay people, of whom there are many in China, will know enough to decide whether they want to start studying it themselves.

I have to keep on reminding myself to remember what we take for granted in our approach to our practice and what my Chinese students have found so intriguingly different. And here the word 'compassion' springs to my mind whenever I think of their surprise. What represents the warmth and closeness of my relationship with my patients is something that they find surprising and, in many ways disturbing.

One of my students asked, 'But how will I learn to deal with my patients' emotions?' Our approach is so different from the standard TCM approach they have been taught at acupuncture college. What they find most surprising is what we as five element acupuncturists take for granted, which is that we are there to support our patients emotionally.

In the West, with our years of emphasis (over-emphasis some of us would say) on self-development and 'finding our inner you', it comes as a surprise when we encounter cultures where introspection of this kind is a luxury or even frowned upon. So not only do Chinese students have to learn the technical aspect of five element acupuncture, they have also to make a major emotional re-adjustment inside themselves as they approach a practice which demands empathy as the most important quality in a therapist.

And if all goes well, and I am happy with the course, I may well think if publishing it in English, too! There are many people all over the world, and not just in China, if the readers of this blog is anything to go by, who may be interested in learning more, and who have no access to any kind of five element teaching.

◇◇◇◇◇◇◇◇◇

17 JANUARY 2013
Beware of the incorrect use of junction points!

I have recently noticed that practitioners are increasingly choosing to use the junction points of an element's two officials together as a matter of course, for example VII (GB) 37 with VIII (Liv) 5 for the Wood element, much as they might choose the paired source or tonification points. I don't know when or why this started to be common practice, but it was certainly not the case during my own training.

It's good to think what the function of a junction point is. What is it actually joining to what? What it does is provide a link between the paired yin and yang officials, drawing energy from one to the other. What happens when we needle VII 37 and VIII 5 together is that we are just drawing energy from Liver to Gall Bladder by tonifying VII 37, and from Gall Bladder to Liver by tonifying VIII 5. But there is only a point to doing this if one or other official is relatively deficient compared with the other. This does not seem to be the reasoning behind the current and growing use of junction points. Usually, the yin and yang officials share their energy and balance any discrepancy without help from us. To draw energy away from one official to the other through their junction points as a matter of course without first considering whether either official needs this support therefore appears to me to be wrong, and may well be a waste of a treatment. And we should never waste treatments.

At an advanced training course with JR, I remember how cross he became when somebody suggested the junction points of Three Heater and Heart Protector as a choice of points for a Fire patient. JR said, 'Are you choosing these because you really think that this patient needs his Inner and Outer Frontier Gates opened, or just because you can't think of any other points?' He said he would choose them only if he felt that the gates were blocked between the two officials. The only other junction points I ever heard him selecting together in all the years that I observed him with patients were those of Stomach and Spleen, XI 40 and XII 4, and he explained that he chose these, not because they happened also to be junction points, but because of the spirit of what each point gave the other.

There are, however, some rare cases when there might be inequality between the yin and yang officials, which needs correcting and which will appear as what is called a split pulse. In all my years of practice, the only time I have found a marked discrepancy of this kind, and used the junction points to treat it, was in a patient who had had a colostomy bag fitted, and whose Lung pulse was markedly much stronger than his Large Intestine pulse. Here I tonified the junction point of the LI, X (LI) 6, to draw the excess energy from the Lung. The Lung and Large Intestine pulses returned to balance with one another, and the patient immediately felt better.

We also use junction points when we want to correct an Akabane imbalance, but this time we draw energy to the same official from one side of the body to the other, not to or from its paired official. And of course they can be used individually for what we call 'their spirit', for example III (Bl) 58 or I (Ht) 5, where my choice will be based upon their name and what I think this point therefore offers its official.

So I would plead with all five element acupuncturists to think carefully about their reasoning for choosing paired junction points. They should ask themselves whether they are simply choosing them because they can't think of anything else to do! If that is the case, then choose the source points, or, if there is enough energy in the mother element, the tonification points. These are points which can be repeated again and again. But to keep on choosing junction points is like keeping on trying to open a door which is already open.

◇◇◇◇◇◇◇◇

18 JANUARY 2013

How clearly an element reveals itself if we have eyes to see

Every day I receive confirmation that the elements do indeed imprint a personal stamp upon each one of us in the shape of one of the five elements. It is both exhilarating and humbling to receive these continuing proofs of the truth of what I practise. I received one such confirmation at a fellow acupuncturist's practice a few days ago, when I was asked to help a patient of hers.

A few years ago this patient had suddenly begun to experience severe pains down his body, accompanied by strange involuntary jerking movements of his left leg. I asked him whether he had been suffering from any particular stresses at the time the pains started, perhaps something which he might experience as a shock to the system. 'No,' he said, but then I noticed his eyes suddenly filling with great sadness. 'Is his element Metal then?', I began to ask myself, as I saw this look of grief. We are always being given pointers to the elements if we are sensitive enough to notice them, however slight they may be, little gifts of help. And then came another gift. He was silent for quite a while as I took his pulses, and then, out of the silence, unexpectedly said quietly, 'I always wished I had had some relationship with my father.' Aha, I thought, who but Metal would say this in this way? For of course Metal has a particular association with the father.

Metal is the 'if only' element, the element that looks back into the past, and often thinks more about this past than about the present. So here was a double pointer to Metal, the grief in the eyes and the immediate connection with a father who, though still living, is as though lost to him.

So I continued with my questioning, guiding it now along a path that my experience tells me that Metal will accept. It wants to be left alone to make its own connections and assess for itself what is relevant or irrelevant. So I suggested lightly that maybe something had indeed happened around the time all this pain appeared. 'Maybe some stress at home or at work, perhaps? But only you will know what that might be.' And I added, 'Perhaps the involuntary jerking of your leg is because you want to kick somebody!' We both laughed, and then he was given his first treatment on Metal, just the source points, and I left him with this rather light, almost joking remark hanging in the air.

A few hours later he phoned, and wanted to tell us both something he had never told anybody else before. Two years ago his wife had had an affair with his best friend, which had devastated him. They had worked through this now, but he could not forgive his friend, and never wanted to see him again – another great loss in his life. I suspect that now that he has admitted to his anger, he will no longer unconsciously need to kick out, either at his wife, or more likely at his friend, as good treatment focused on his Metal element helps him gradually heal.

This was further evidence for me that we need only lightly suggest something to Metal, and then stand back to allow them space to work out their own solutions, since Metal is so acute and quick at making connections for itself.

How much we achieved in such a short time!

I'm sure five element acupuncturists reading this will expect me to write about any other sensory signs of Metal I noticed. His emotion I have talked about, his colour was not very clearly what I associate with Metal. I couldn't detect any smell at all, but the sound of his voice was very flat, very yin, dragging me down with it. This is the sound which I associate with Metal's weeping tone.

◇◇◇◇◇◇◇◇

21 JANUARY 2013

Announcing the pending publication of my Teach Yourself Five Element Acupuncture for Acupuncturists*

The ideal introduction to a healing discipline such as five element acupuncture is in the form of a personal transmission from master to pupil. This was the only way people learned in the past, where the handing down of experience from one generation of a family to the next was common practice and the only type of learning available. Modern forms of education, though, have increasingly emphasized the need to gather students together into classrooms, there to follow rigidly standardized courses with a ratio of one tutor to a roomful of students. It is little wonder, then, that against this backdrop of formalized learning, the transmission of many years of deeply personal experiences from a practitioner to a student is a luxury denied to all but the very lucky few, those ones who have been able to find a teacher whose teachings they admire and who lives close enough to them to be available at sufficiently regular intervals to pass on his/her knowledge.

This being so sadly the case now, and the situation being made even harder by the lack of good five element clinicians prepared to teach, I have decided to do what I can to fill a

---

* Now forming an appendix to the revised edition of my *Handbook of Five Element Practice* (Singing Dragon, 2014).

glaring gap by writing this manual based upon my *Handbook of Five Element Practice*. Since I cannot single-handedly (or with just a few other five element teachers) satisfy the growing need for this kind of personal transmission of what I have learnt, then I hope this manual will provide something which I cannot offer in any other way. The purist will complain that long-distance learning of this kind is not only far from ideal but perhaps should not even be undertaken, because the student can be given so little feedback. But the purist is not confronted, as I am, with many hundreds of Chinese acupuncturists from all over their vast country longing to learn about five element acupuncture, and many more spread all over the world, eagerly learning whatever they can through this blog.

For Chinese and other non-English-speaking students there are the additional problems of language barriers which complicate communication, both written and verbal. Hence the eventual appearance of these lessons in both a Mandarin version for my Chinese students and an English version for all those other people of different nationalities, equally keen to learn, if the numbers reading my blog are anything to go by, and for whom English must be their lingua franca.

The Mandarin version of this self-tuition course is being translated by Mei Long as I write, so that it will be available for our next seminar in Nanning in April 2013. I am just completing the English version, which I am planning to issue in book form. I have yet to decide whether I will also include a kind of addendum listing the (very few) points I use and my reasoning for using them. This is something I am working on at the moment.

◇◇◇◇◇◇◇◇◇

4 FEBRUARY 2013
Further thoughts on Water

I pass on some further insights about the Water element which have come to me this morning all the way from India from a Water friend of mine who is very perceptive about her own element:

'Water can be aggressive. It's more a wearing-down kind of persistent aggression rather than periodic pushes (as Wood might do) but it's always easier to analyze in retrospect. Aggression generally brings out reactions in the observer, which throw him/her off balance and make it harder to figure out what is happening.

I have put up on my fridge door a reminder of the three fearlessnesses (from Lao Tzu), which are:

The fearlessness of taking pain

The fearlessness to suffer loss

The fearlessness towards ferocity'

Thank you for these thoughts, Sujata!

◇◇◇◇◇◇◇◇◇

22 FEBRUARY 2013
The results of two simple treatments

I am always happy to receive confirmation of how effective five element acupuncture can be, and particularly so if this comes from my own treatment. Yesterday I had the simplest of treatments, the clearing of a XII/I (Spleen/Heart) Entry/Exit block finishing with the source points of the Small Intestine and Heart. I slept better, leaping out of bed without for once thinking I needed to stretch my poor old knees to get them working, as I usually have to. I interpret the clarity of my thoughts and the increased mobility of my body to the release of the blocked energy in the Earth element, particularly the Spleen, the transporter of energy round the body.

The second happy result from treatment was told me yesterday by a fellow acupuncturist. A patient of his came for her first treatment for a distressing skin condition covering the whole of one arm with a large red rash which not even prolonged steroid treatment had managed to control. He diagnosed her as being Fire, did the usual Aggressive Energy drain, plus the source points of Outer Fire. She rang to tell him that her skin had reacted quite strongly the next day, but by the morning of the second day the rash had disappeared completely, leaving both her and her acupuncturist amazed at the speed of change.

Long live simple five element treatment! Who dares still say that you can't treat physical symptoms with it?

24 FEBRUARY 2013

Acupuncture and herbs: a five element approach

In my first year at acupuncture college JR Worsley explained to us his decision not to incorporate a study of herbs into the curriculum. This was because 'herbology', as he called it, was such a profound discipline that it required as many years of study as acupuncture, and, like the food we should be eating, the herbs prescribed should come from the country in which we are living.

I have since thought a lot about this, and added my own understanding as to why I think acupuncture, or five element acupuncture in particular, needs to stand alone as a discipline. In acupuncture we work from the inside out, stimulating a patient's own energy back to health and relying only on this energy to do the work. Herbs, on the other hand, are foreign substances entering the body from the outside, and have a different action. To offer both herbs and acupuncture is therefore, to me, a bit like a Pushmi-pullyu approach (a two-headed animal familiar to me from my childhood reading of Doctor Doolittle), as though we may be tugging a patient's energies in different directions. And, even if I considered it necessary, which I don't, I certainly haven't had available to me the years of study required to reach a competent level equivalent to that of my study of acupuncture.

Interestingly, Liu Lihong, my host in China, and an outstandingly skilled herbalist of many years' standing, has told my students, all of them originally also herbalists, not to practise both, but to concentrate entirely on acupuncture.

This blog has been prompted by questions from a fellow practitioner who had heard a herbalist 'who also does acupuncture' talking about the need always to add herbs to acupuncture for infertility treatment. Many herbalists do a bit of acupuncture, as many acupuncturists feel they should add a few herbs, but in my view you can't add little snippets of other disciplines into your practice without confusing the elements and, as a five element acupuncturist, that is the last thing you want to do.

◇◇◇◇◇◇◇◇

27 FEBRUARY 2013

Treating a patient with terminal lung cancer

Today I received this very moving email from a practitioner who has come to my seminars. She is happy for me to pass on what she has written because, she told me, 'like yourself, I am keen to share experiences so that others may glean a little knowledge which may help them in future treatments'. So here is what she has told me:

'I am writing to share with you my experience so far of treating my patient with terminal cancer, where, without your guidance and influence, and your mantra of "the simpler, the better" I feel I would not have been able to do my best.

(When I saw this patient for the first time) he was complaining of severe abdominal pain, had lost a huge amount of weight and was now having difficulty breathing. A&E had been pumping him full of morphine and then discharging him within hours of admission. In the first two treatments I was able to carry out IDs, AE drain and source points for Wood, after which he said he felt energized and went out for his first walk in months. He cancelled his third treatment as he was admitted into hospital for chest x-rays and investigations (finally), whereupon it emerged that he has a very aggressive form of lung cancer (secondary), with the primary suspected in the large intestine. He started chemotherapy there and then, but expressed a wish to carry on with his acupuncture treatments as soon as he was able.

Just after I saw you last at Guy's Clinical Skills Day earlier this month, I was reading your book *The Pattern of Things** on the train on the journey home, and came upon the very moving chapter describing your treatment of Martine just before she died. This was a very poignant moment for me as it was whilst I was reading this that I received a text message telling me of my patient's diagnosis and asking whether I would be willing to treat him in hospital, to which I agreed, thankful for the strength and insight I had gained from reading your piece.

… I was finally able to see him in the hospice today. I had mentally planned my treatment – AE again, possibly H/W, possibly Rich for the Vitals (Bl 38 (43)) or Kidney chest points – only to be told that I wasn't to put needles in his chest or back, and to be honest, he is now so emaciated that I would have been a tad fearful to do so (even the muscles either side of his spine had disappeared to nothing). He was barely able to talk because of the breathlessness, and his pulses were non-existent except in the Lu/LI position. I contemplated H/W but thought him to be too weak to tolerate that many needles, so in the end I did source points in one foot only, which sent him off to sleep for half an hour or so.

As an ex-asthmatic myself, I know how incredibly tense my back used to get during an attack and so I offered to gently massage his back, which he was very grateful for, and proceeded to massage neck, shoulders, arms, hands and feet for about an hour. He was visibly more relaxed afterwards and

---

*   Now published as *Patterns of Practice* (Singing Dragon, 2014).

his breathing had become much less laboured, and so at this point I took my leave.

My apologies for the lengthy prose here, but I will finish now by thanking you, Nora, for instilling in me the courage to do less in order to do more, and to carry out my treatments with utmost humility.'

I think this is a good summary of an excellent approach to helping the terminally ill. (The only thing I suggested was that there would have been no need to worry about clearing a H/W, because clearing it reduces the stress on the Heart, which can only be helpful.)

◇◇◇◇◇◇◇◇

7 MARCH 2013
Update on the patient with lung cancer

(See my blog of 27 February 2013.)

Here is what the practitioner has just emailed me:

'My patient continues to amaze me! I saw him again today – day 3 after his second round of chemo – he looks, sounds and feels extremely well and positive, with very few side effects from all the drugs, save some quite extreme mood swings for the first couple of days immediately after the chemo. His lungs have remained free from fluid and his abdominal pain has subsided, so he is now able to sleep almost horizontally instead of in the upright position which he has had to adopt continually for the past three months or so.

Pulses showed a significant improvement in the Ht/SI position, with a modicum in the Bl/Ki position. Lu/LI was still dominant by far, and I could also detect a very small amount of energy in the other two right-hand positions. The guardian element (Wood) is still very much depleted however.

I repeated H/W today and finished on source points of Wood again, and left it at that. He always falls into a very deep sleep during treatment and for a short while afterwards, and wakes feeling very calm and relaxed.

And I continue to feel humbled by the effects of such a simple treatment, made so much more powerful by the patient himself in choosing to fight to live.'

Well done, Jo!

◇◇◇◇◇◇◇◇

8 MARCH 2013
There is no place for arrogance in the practice room

I was looking at a patient with a class of students recently, and after ten minutes talking to the patient in front of the class I asked them if anybody had seen, heard, (smelt!) or felt anything which pointed to a particular element. One of them said, 'Well it's obviously Fire.' This gave me a jolt, because it reminded me how I, too, at this student's stage of learning, had often thought that a patient's element was obvious, only to find with surprise that I had got it quite wrong. It is the word 'obviously' that a five element acupuncturist must avoid at all costs, because no element will ever be obvious to even the most experienced acupuncturist after a mere ten minutes. We can so easily fall into a trap of relying upon stereotypes of different elements we have formulated for ourselves, and sticking to them through thick and thin, only to find out later on how wrong we have been. (The element proved not to be Fire, either!)

We should always respect the mystery which lies deep within another human being, and which the elements express in all their subtlety. Learning to fathom this mystery can never be a matter of a mere few minutes' superficial interaction.

Nothing about our practice can ever be described as dealing with the obvious. We deal with the not-obvious, however challenging this may be. And this is why I love what I do.

◇◇◇◇◇◇◇◇

11 MARCH 2013
Learning to build up a good relationship with our patients

Like all skills, we have to practise how to create a good relationship with our patients. A successful relationship is one where we are able to make as smooth a match as possible between what we have to offer and what our patients need. Here, of course, our knowledge of the elements will act as our guide, for what one person needs will differ very markedly from what somebody of a different element will need. Some people are lucky, and either by their nature or by the circumstance of their lives have an ability to empathize with other people that a fellow practitioner has first to learn, and all of us will find it easier dealing with some elements than with others. Perhaps to some people's surprise we are not necessarily most at our ease with those of our own element, because seeing our own needs reflected in a patient may make it difficult for us to maintain an appropriate distance. The secret here is to recognize that we may always find certain relationships with our patients more complex and difficult than others, and remain aware of this as we engage with these patients.

I will describe some of my own reactions and difficulties with patients of certain elements (see the following blogs). These are personal to me, and every other practitioner must study their own responses and learn from them. But learn they must, otherwise they will not understand their patients' needs. More importantly their patients will not feel understood, and then their elements will take to hiding themselves away. How can a five element acupuncturist treat if we don't know which element is crying out for help?

Nobody should think that this comes easily to any of us. When I look back at my own practice, I can see many instances where I did not understand what a patient needed, and I offered my help in a way which was not wanted. Inevitably it was these patients who decided quite quickly that I was not the practitioner for them. And they were right! How could I help somebody if I was misreading what they were asking of me? It was as though I was talking in an emotional language foreign to these patients, or rather assuming that both of us were talking in the same language when we very obviously were not. One way of looking at relationships with our patients is thus to see them as though they require us to learn to speak in an emotional language with which only our patient is familiar and at ease in. We therefore need to learn to speak in a different emotional language for each patient. And like learning any new language, this takes time and a good deal of practice.

We all know the warm feeling we have when we have got it right with a patient. It is those times when we know that we have not which we should accept as teaching us the most. JR always said that it was far better if students observing him with patients did not get the elements he diagnosed right, because the only true learning is through our mistakes.

◇◇◇◇◇◇◇◇

11 MARCH 2013
Learning to build up a good relationship with Wood and Fire patients

If I look at my relationship with the Wood element, as my first example, I realize that it has taken me a long time to work out a way of dealing with its strong needs. I tend to go through almost the same pattern of behaviour each time I encounter a Wood patient. I pass through an initial period of wanting to step away, as though shrinking from the push I feel coming towards me, then I experience a flicker, or more than a flicker, of irritation at feeling that I am being outmanoeuvred in some way, before I finally reach a more balanced stage of understanding where I know that to help my Wood patient I have to stand firm and, as it were, counter-punch, however gently.

With all Fire patients, on the other hand, I experience first a slight feeling of relief, since I am moving on to the familiar territory of my own element, accompanied by an initial sense of relaxation. Fire is the most articulate of all elements, enjoying speech as its way of communicating. Since I, too, like communicating through speech, it is easy for the patient and me to fall into the habit of indulging in a kind of idle chatter with which we both feel at ease. Experience has taught me, though, that I must issue a warning to myself to take care and not let the ease of this interaction divert from the reason why the patient is here. I have to be aware, too, that in its need to make other people happy, Fire may also feel it should make light of its problems, and I have to be on the look-out in case I buy into the cheerful mask and ignore what lies beneath it.

One way I have devised of helping me here is through the simple expedient of employing silence, a tool we too seldom use in the practice room. I try consciously to quieten the emotional tone by reminding myself to fall silent. Silence on my part gives my patient permission to stop any superficial chatter, and offers them the space to think out what they really need to tell me. I have often found falling silent is the most difficult thing for me to do, and I have had to train myself to be on the alert against encouraging a babble of words to flood the practice room.

Although it is easy for me to develop a very warm relationship with all my Fire patients, this ironically makes it harder to set the correct emotional tone which is helpful for my patients. Familiarity does not breed contempt, far from it in this case, but it certainly breeds a false sense of relaxation.

◇◇◇◇◇◇◇◇◇

12 MARCH 2013
Learning to build up a good relationship with Earth patients

The difficulties I experience with Earth patients are of a different kind from those with Wood or Fire. I have found that the need to be nurtured which all Earth people have awakes an echo of the same need in me, because at some deep level within me I would like some of the same kind of nurturing I am being asked to offer Earth. A few days ago, interestingly, an Earth practitioner told me that he finds his first interaction with his patients disturbing because he feels their differing needs tugging at his Earth element, which is reluctant to offer what is being demanded of it.

Once I am aware of this reaction in myself, I remind myself firmly that I am here for the patient and not for my own needs. What Earth needs is not a blanket response of sympathy of the 'Oh, you poor dear' kind, but instead it needs to be understood. It wants to be heard, and wants to be heard to the end if possible without interruption. Its thinking is a circular process, ending where it began and then beginning again. If it is out of balance, it begins again with the same words and goes over the same ground, like an oxen tied to a circular grindstone, going round and round. When it is in balance, this need to churn over the same thoughts is lessened, but never disappears completely. Since its function is to process all things, thoughts as well as food, it has to perform this task endlessly as the other elements pass their energies to it for processing.

If I remain clear that my Earth patients need to be allowed time to circle round a subject, even though I may have heard the same thing in the same words before, I am able to stand back and allow this circular movement to continue without getting irritated. But being a quick thinker and talker myself, the slow chewing-of-the-cud which is Earth's way of thinking can tend to irritate me and make me want to interrupt it if I am not careful. So a warning sign goes off in my head with every Earth patient I treat: Let the patient speak, Nora, and only interrupt or add your own comments when you have given your patient time to process his/her thoughts and express them fully in the way they want.

◇◇◇◇◇◇◇◇◇

12 MARCH 2013
Learning to build up a good relationship with Metal and Water patients

With Metal I seem to have a far less difficult relationship than with the other elements, perhaps because it demands space to be itself and allows me time to catch my breath, as it were. No immediate reaction is demanded of me, except an acceptance that it wants to be the judge of how our relationship should develop in a way satisfactory to itself. It is happy with space and is the most comfortable of all the elements with silence, for it needs silence in which to work out its own solutions to life's problems. This need for space and silence offers a great challenge to my Fire element, if I do not recognize it in time, and find myself starting to gabble to fill the silence. With all Metal patients I have learnt, too, that I must hold back my own impulse to share my thoughts, for this can easily lead to a kind of role reversal since I find that I can often learn from Metal's detached wisdom.

Metal patients are not, however, there to teach me, nor for me to teach them, but to find the support for their Metal energies which treatment will offer them. With Metal I need almost say nothing and let the treatment do its work silently. The practice of silence which Metal needs is that which respects its need to solve its own problems. The silence which I have to encourage myself to offer Fire is different; it is aimed at preventing it from talking so much that it forgets why it is coming for treatment.

Finally I come to the problems I may experience in dealing appropriately with my Water patients. I do not find the demands Water makes upon me difficult to meet, although others may. The need for a reassuring approach to still the panic which lies deep within the heart of all Water people is not something alien to me, but something I feel at ease with and able to offer without feeling in any way diminished, as I may do with Earth.

My main difficulty comes from my inability to recognize the Water element in my patients quickly enough in the first place. We all know how Water likes to disguise itself and hide, and it has taken me longer to detect its presence than that of the other elements. Even now I have a tendency to see Water's uneasy laughter as coming from Fire. Its elusive nature will often make me question whether I am really in the presence of Water or not. Once recognized, though, I feel able to offer what I think it needs, provided that I stay focused on the profound fears which lie beneath its often apparently confident surface. This most ambitious of all elements, and the one most likely to get to the top of whatever profession it chooses, harbours a terrified underbelly. I must never overlook its need for these hidden fears to be acknowledged by me, and for me to offer them the correct level of reassurance.

Readers will have noticed that where possible I like to write about interesting experiences other practitioners tell me about. The blogs about the treatment of a patient with lung cancer illustrate why I find this so important. The more that is written about the practice of five element acupuncture the more those reading about it will learn through others' experiences as much as they can through their own. And the more encouragement they will get for their own practice.

◇◇◇◇◇◇◇◇

25 MARCH 2013

Latest update from the practitioner treating the patient with lung cancer

(See my blogs of 27 February and 7 March 2013.)

I have just received this heartening update from the practitioner:

'Just thought I'd update you briefly – I have continued to visit my patient twice weekly in the Hospice and he is going from strength to strength, despite a major setback a couple of weeks ago. At that time, he had been doing very well indeed – he was no longer reliant upon oxygen, his breathing was normal, had good pain control and had regained his appetite. In acupuncture terms, H/W had cleared and I was treating him very minimally, purely on command points. However, things went pear-shaped a couple of days later when his bowels appeared to be blocked – he was eating an enormous amount of food (2500 calories per day) but his bowels had stopped working (probably due to the morphine and other drugs) and nothing was getting through. He was once again in tremendous pain, had a stomach drain in situ, was nil by mouth and was scheduled to have ileostomy surgery. H/W had returned with a vengeance, he was in very low spirits and did not feel up to any needling, so I treated the H/W with acupressure instead.

A few days later, I received a message that his bowels had started to work again and that he had a reprieve from surgery – and when could I come to give him another treatment! At my next visit, once again I was amazed at the difference in him – H/W had disappeared again, and the pulses were the most even to date. This time I cleared AE and finished on source points.

I am due to see him again today and he is due to go home on Wednesday all being well, though he will be continuing with his chemotherapy as an outpatient. He feels that the work we are doing together is extremely worthwhile and really looks forward to his treatments, as he says he feels very focused and strong afterwards, and also relaxed and rested, but energized. Above all, he says I'm probably his only visitor who comes without making any demands, physically or emotionally – for which he is immensely grateful.

This experience brings home to me how important it is to be aware of our own emotions and to maintain a balance, especially through difficult times, where words can be superfluous – a mere presence is enough.'

I cannot praise this practitioner enough for the courage to keep things simple and not panic. As I wrote to her in reply to this email:

'It is never easy to treat somebody who is so ill. There will always be times when their health deteriorates suddenly, as their body struggles to cope both with the disease and with the side-effects of the drastic treatment they are getting. But you seem really to be helping him.

I love what he said about you being "probably the only visitor who comes without making any demands, physically or emotionally". You can't have a better compliment!'

Nor can you have a better illustration of the rare quality we all need to nurture in ourselves as practitioners, and, too, as human beings, not to make demands, either physical or emotional, upon those around us which they are unable to meet.

◇◇◇◇◇◇◇◇◇

27 MARCH 2013

Trying not to cast our own shadows over our patients

Yesterday I caught myself talking to a patient about something personal to me, prompted by what the patient was telling me. As I said it, I realized that I had made a mistake, for I could feel that my remark had slightly changed the direction of what the patient wanted to tell me. It was as if I had interposed my shadow between the patient and me.

I have often said that we should try to cast as few of our own shadows over those we encounter, because these distort our relationships with them. This is particularly true of our encounters with our patients, where the need for maturity on the practitioner's part is at its greatest. For if we utter an unwise remark or react clumsily, our patient will feel constrained to adapt his/her behaviour, however slightly, to take account of what appears to be a problematic area they perceive in us, and may well hesitate to open themselves up further. Then the chance for them to feel free to explain themselves without inhibition may be lost, and our relationship with them may descend into the kind of superficial encounter which characterizes much of everyday life.

The practice room should not reflect such superficialities. It should be the place where the patient feels free not to have to adapt their behaviour to take their practitioner's personal needs into account. As practitioners we have to learn to remain true to ourselves, whilst assessing with each patient how far it is appropriate to share some of our personal views, but never to burden them with our problems.

◇◇◇◇◇◇◇◇◇

23 APRIL 2013
Back from my fourth visit to Nanning

What to say about this fourth visit? Each has been so different and each has added a further layer to the foundation of five element acupuncture which we are gradually building on Chinese soil. We have now reached the point where some of our first students are themselves feeling confident enough to start giving some simple introductory classes to new groups of acupuncturists. Altogether we had a total of just over 60 students, of whom about 25 had come to previous seminars. I will try and download the group photo of all of us in front of the Nanning Centre.

This was the first time I had two other tutors with me, Mei Long and Guy Caplan. I was happy to hand over the more structured teaching of five element clinical skills to Guy, which left Mei and me more time to concentrate on looking after the many people who wanted treatment.

Mei had already sent over her translation of my *Teach Yourself Five Element Acupuncture* manual. This was printed during our visit, and copies given to each class member. The manual contains 16 lessons based upon my *Handbook of Five Element Practice*, and offers a step-by-step introduction to five element diagnosis and treatment protocols. This will be a great help for those students who have no access whatsoever to any five element teaching apart from their brief few weeks with us.

We have decided that at our next seminar in the autumn we will concentrate on the group of practitioners who are already practising five element acupuncture to help them become more confident in their skills. It is intended that this group will form the basis of a future five element teaching team spread across China, the declared aim of Liu Lihong, our host and the director of the Nanning Centre.

I had felt rather discouraged about my Mandarin studies before I left for China, but to my surprise, I discovered that I must be learning more than I realize. I could perceive sentence structures better, although I definitely haven't yet got a large enough vocabulary to make myself understood. I found myself, though, fumbling around for a few words, and, with much sign language and smiles, I managed occasionally to make myself understood. So that is at least a tiny step forward. Gratifyingly, many of the students are determined to learn more English so that they can talk to us, and certainly their English has much improved. So I will go back to my Mandarin classes with greater enthusiasm now.

Finally, Guy and I had our own mini-adventure during an overnight stay in Chengdu on the way back. We were caught up in the after-shock of the Sichuan earthquake as we had our breakfast on the 30th floor of the hotel. The restaurant shook violently for a moment or so, and the guests looked around at each other unsure what to do. Eventually, a door to the emergency stairs was opened, and we started to climb down steep, narrow concrete steps in pitch darkness. We were later told that the hotel staff should have told us just to wait for the tremors to stop, which is what those in Chengdu do, since they are used to these shocks and take no notice of them.

Luckily Guy had a torch on his i-phone and lighted the way for me as I stumbled down step after step from the 30th to the 21st floor. There, to our amusement, we discovered that there had been no emergency in the rest of the hotel. All was as normal, as we emerged onto the hotel corridor to find other guests going quietly about their business unaware of the adventure we had been through. We went to our rooms, leaving behind the other people in our group presumably still stumbling on down the concrete well for a further 21 flights to the ground floor.

◇◇◇◇◇◇◇◇

27 MAY 2013

Two humbling experiences

I have been very humbled by two experiences I have had in the last month or so, one as I left China, and the other on my return. Both are heart-warming reminders to me of how fortunate I am to do what I do.

My Chinese experience came on the last day of my stay in Nanning. My host, Liu Lihong, wanted to find out how each of the 60 students who had attended our two weeks of seminars had found them. So we asked each one in turn to tell us. What astounded me, and I hope pleased Liu Lihong, was the group's unanimous expression of overwhelming delight in what they had learnt and how amazed they were at the compassion and understanding we showed the many patients whose treatments they observed. This was a facet of practice apparently totally new to them, and opened a fresh window for them onto the importance of developing a warm patient/ practitioner relationship.

My other example, from the other side of the world here in London, illustrates just this important aspect of our practice. It comes in an email from the practitioner who has been telling me of her experience in treating a terminally ill cancer patient over the last few months of his life, and how profound an effect this has had on her (see my three previous blogs on 27 February, 7 March and 25 March 2013).

Although she was sad to have to report her patient's death, she sees her time with him in the most positive light. With her permission, I give below her description of what the experience has meant to her:

'The past months since his diagnosis in January this year have been a real roller coaster for him, both physically and emotionally. Things took a dramatic turn for the worse last Wednesday and I feel so relieved that his suffering and strife were not prolonged further and that he is now truly at peace.

I feel very privileged to have been invited into this person's life. His very obvious Wood CF was very refreshing to me, though not without its challenges to his nearest and dearest. His thirst for information about his treatments and acupuncture as a whole was a delight and not at all threatening to me – he was extremely open to the whole Chinese medicine ethos and it could be said that he was rather unorthodox in his beliefs and actions, and extremely proud of the fact he was too!

His openness, honesty and need for straight talking could have easily come across as slightly abrasive, but for me it made the whole subject of cancer and death very accessible. At a time when some would feel the need to avoid or skirt around what is a very difficult subject, I felt able to talk candidly to him without fear of overstepping the mark or holding back, in order to say what needed to be said.

You have often said, Nora, how you learn so much from your patients. My relationship with this patient has been a very emotional, memorable and powerful lesson – but most of all, very humbling indeed.'

As with my patient Martine, about whom I wrote in the last chapter of my *Pattern of Things*, experiences such as those this practitioner had to learn to deal with touch us at the deepest level. They leave us much changed, and by this change open us up to greater understanding of the needs of our patients.

Both these experiences, from different parts of the world, remind me once again of the common thread which runs through all of us. Whatever tribe, race, country or continent we come from, the five great fingers of the elements hold each of us in their grasp, shaping the deepest aspects of ourselves and giving us a common humanity.

✧✧✧✧✧✧✧✧✧

26 MAY 2013
One of the burdens of being Inner Fire

Oh, the ridiculous unnecessary pressures my Small Intestine official can put me under!

Yesterday I travelled by train to Salisbury, not something requiring much mental exertion, one would think. But with every train journey I take comes the moment as I walk along the platform when I have to decide whether I want to head for the carriage with the quiet zone, and opt for a journey theoretically free of people talking loudly on their mobiles, or just sit in an ordinary carriage and suffer. As everybody now probably knows, I absolutely hate mobile phones, however necessary they have become, not only because of the complete disregard for other people their owners show, but also because they are increasingly cutting people physically off from contact with one another – ironically, because they are intended to do just the opposite. So do I suffer a journey interrupted by the endless pinging of mobile phones, and forced to listen to conversations I have absolutely no interest in, or do I sit in a carriage in peaceful silence?

Except it is rarely silent, I have found. What usually happens is that somebody, finding that there are more seats available than elsewhere, plonks themselves down without seeing where they are sitting, and immediately switches on their phone. Then there comes the moment when I look round to see if any other occupant is as annoyed as I am, which they, surprisingly, rarely are. So I am forced yet again to gesture to the signs on the window, to be greeted usually, not by an apology, but by irritation, with the speaker either hurriedly grabbing his/her bags to walk to another carriage or walking through the carriage to the area beyond the door still talking loudly.

And this may happen not once but twice during a journey. And if it doesn't happen, then at every station along the route, as new passengers come in, I tense myself for another such encounter. What an utter waste of my energy! Wouldn't it be far better for me, plagued as I am with bad hearing, just to turn off both hearing aids and sit in utter silence wherever I choose? But I know that when I take my next train journey, I will go through the same rigmarole.

It is on occasions like this that I would love to be any other element than Inner Fire to allow my poor Small Intestine simply to relax and enjoy the journey, rather wasting so much time sorting things out in such an unsatisfactory way. But, sadly I often think, it can never truly relax, as it sifts and sorts, sifts and sorts to protect the Heart.

◇◇◇◇◇◇◇◇

4 JUNE 2013
My approach to pulse-taking

I have been privileged to receive from Peter Eckman a draft of his latest book, which is about pulses and is about to be published, like mine, by Singing Dragon. I love its title, *The Compleat Acupuncturist: A Guide to Constitutional and Conditional Pulse Diagnosis*, an echo of Isaak Walton's *The Compleat Angler* (1653). The book discusses in great detail the many, many different ways in which pulses are taken and the many, many different ways in which they are interpreted.

This has set me thinking about my own approach to pulse-taking, best summed up, I feel, by something I said to those attending my last SOFEA clinical seminar. In effect I told them, a bit tongue in cheek, to 'forget the pulses'. This is something I often find myself saying to practitioners in an attempt to remove some of the unnecessary burden they feel when trying to interpret pulses. I suggest, instead, that they should concentrate on looking at the patient as a whole whose pulses are only one of many manifestations of the elements. I always labour the point that the extreme subtlety of what these 12 pulses are telling us makes their interpretation an art which has to be honed over many years, and like all arts is a skill that is never perfected.

My approach is based upon what I was taught as an undergraduate at Leamington, where the importance of pulse-taking was never over-emphasized. We were told simply to take as many pulses as we could (100 a month, if I remember correctly), and gradually learn to assess the strengths and weaknesses of the different pulses in relation to one another. The aim was mainly to detect energy blocks, such as Entry/Exit blocks or those occurring in a Husband/Wife imbalance. It was firmly drilled into us that pulses never told us what the guardian element (CF) was, because even if treatment was directed at the right element, it might well be this element's pulses which showed the least response to treatment because of its role in shepherding the other elements into balance.

The famous 27 pulse qualities were only mentioned once by JR, almost as an aside, when, as part of what was apparently considered necessary to complete the syllabus, he raced through the different pulse qualities in about 15 minutes with obvious disinterest, ending with telling us, 'and that's all you need to know about the 27 pulses qualities'. This appeared to be a doorway through which he did not think it necessary for us to pass.

Another occasion with JR had a much more profound effect on me. I told him at one point that sometimes I felt that I couldn't interpret anything my fingers were trying to tell me. He said, 'I know what you mean. I will feel the same, and then perhaps a month later I will realize that my pulse-taking has moved to another level.'

These words of his hover over my fingers as I take pulses even now. I never wait too long to try and interpret what I feel, and can even find myself talking as I take them, almost as if I want to allow my mind to do its thinking through words so that it sets my spirit free just to feel. And then I try to add what I am feeling to what my other senses are telling me to help me interpret the signals the patients is sending me through everything they do or say.

What worries me about approaches to pulse-taking is that pulses represent one of the few aspects of five element practice where we ask for a physical response from a patient's body. All the other forms of diagnosis are much more ephemeral. We can't physically touch a smell, a sound of voice, a colour or an emotion, but we can certainly physically touch a hand to feel a pulse. And the physical appears to provide a reassuring refuge to which we can retreat if our other senses confuse us and prove too elusive. I have decided that this is the reason why all novice practitioners (and quite a few experienced practitioners, too!) immediately reach for the hands of the patient lying there on the couch, rather than paying attention to the patient as a whole, as though needing to anchor themselves immediately in the physical. Sometimes I feel, rather wickedly, that this is a bit like a drowning person grasping a lifebuoy.

Except in the case of blocks, where I always try to add other information to what my fingers may be telling me, pulses play an almost subsidiary role compared with what I learn from the total picture presented by the patient. So Peter and I, both trained in the same school, but he, unlike me, having received much more extensive training in other disciplines, have arrived at somewhat different points on the scale of the importance we attribute to what our fingers can tell us. I am nonetheless fascinated by all those other approaches his new book covers, but which I know I may only ever appreciate in theory, not in practice.

(See also my other two blogs on pulse-taking: *The mystery of pulses*, 22 October 2010, and *Using our two hands*, 24 February 2012.)

Unfortunately my plans for visiting Jacques Lavier's daughter in Toulouse and my two visits to China had to be put on hold because of my illness in July 2013, which jolted the whole remainder of 2013 out of shape. This is the reason for the quite long break in my blogs between 18 June and 30 August.

◇◇◇◇◇◇◇◇

18 JUNE 2013
The rewards of teaching in China

Mei has just forwarded me the following heart-warming email from one of our Chinese students. I am passing on the flavour of what this practitioner said in her own words below:

'Today I treated a CV/GV block, and up the pulses raised! And our heart, me and my patient, was on the wings of joy. Really I can't believe this, that the illness which has made him suffering for years will be indeed conquered by this tiny little needle?

He was very satisfied and his wife even moved to tears. Thank you so much for bringing our old treasure back to home! Such a huge contribution.'

It is lovely for me to see our students over there putting into practice what they have learnt from us, and, as they often tell us, helping so many of their patients to a happier, healthier life. It is such rewarding, worthwhile work. Although I hardly need any more encouragement than I already have, this lovely feedback is further confirmation that what we are teaching falls on very fertile ground.

◇◇◇◇◇◇◇◇

30 AUGUST 2013
Explanation for this gap in my blogs

My readers may have noticed that it has been some time since I posted my last blog here. This was unfortunately forced upon me by an unexpected stay in hospital as a result of a subdural haematoma of the brain. Thankfully I am now much restored, and, to general relief, my brain is apparently unaffected. I have been told that all that hard mental work I have been doing trying to learn Mandarin and updating my books for re-publication by my new publishers has helped to keep my brain active, and has actually benefited my recovery. So roll on my next Mandarin class!

I have been advised, though, to cut back on my travels for the next few months, something I was at first reluctant to agree to, but have now come to see as sensible. So this has brought to a halt my next planned expeditions to Beijing and Nanning for the time being, as well as one or two shorter European trips.

In whatever happens to me I always try to see the lessons life is teaching me. Quite apart from having to deal with the after-effects of my illness on my body, the most difficult thing for me so far has been to acknowledge the fallibility of this body, and accept that I will need to take it increasingly into account as the years pass and weigh more heavily upon it. It has made me aware, too, of how lucky I have so far been with my health, and how fortunate to have managed to do what I have wanted to in relation to my acupuncture work. Most importantly it has given me the opportunity to spread my love of five element acupuncture as widely as I can. More of this in my next blog.

11 SEPTEMBER 2013

How sad that there are now so few pure five element practitioners

What a pity there are so few people now in the UK or elsewhere in the world, it seems, who are just practising five element acupuncture as we were all taught it by JR Worsley. In other words, these are people who base their practice on directing all their efforts at strengthening one element which gives each person their particular direction in life. So many people now, it appears, mix this approach with all kinds of different add-ons, such as Japanese acupuncture, treatment of syndromes, herbs, Tuina or ear acupuncture. Each of these can have their own quite valid approach to balancing a patient's health, but, when added to treatment on the guardian element, dilutes what we are offering by confusing the elements. It's a bit as though we are speaking one language with the elements, and then throw in the odd phrase in another language.

There are not many people now, it appears, who have the courage to attempt to pinpoint a patient's element and then simply strengthen it by working on points on its officials. Perhaps it sounds too simple just to concentrate on an element's command points, with the occasional spirit point added to strengthen it. And, then again, practitioners are often in too much of a hurry to achieve what is realistically much too quick a result, and reach too soon for other tools, instead of waiting and letting the element chosen do its work slowly and steadily.

The more we practise, the more we will find that we will be quick to recognize the subtle changes which take place when a patient's element is fed with what it needs through its own points. It still amazes me how quickly some slight thing about the patient will show an immediate, if sometimes tiny, response to treatment which my senses can perceive in some way – a slight change of colour, a relaxing of tension somewhere in the face, an easier relationship with me. It is as though a different person gradually emerges as they take the tiny steps which lead from imbalance to balance.

So to any practitioner out there attempting to find their way in the profound world of the elements, I will say again, as I have said many times, learn to have the courage to rely on the patient's element to restore health, and give yourself enough time to find that element. Just because JR Worsley, with 50 years of practice, could home in on an element very quickly doesn't mean that we, who have many less years' experience, have to do the same. It always takes time and steady practice finally to be satisfied that we have found that particular patient's element. There is never any need for hurry. Patients are only impatient if they sense our insecurity.

But to end this blog on an optimistic note, how good that there are now hundreds of practitioners in China eager to learn this approach to their practice. I was heartened to hear that one of our Chinese students, now practising five element acupuncture in a very large practice in Beijing, has so impressed people there with the amazing results she is achieving that they are very keen to find more five element practitioners to teach the other acupuncture practitioners there. So the East is now recognizing what the West had started to discard. It is a sad irony, but let us hope the East in its eagerness to attach itself again to its five element roots has again something to teach the West here.

◇◇◇◇◇◇◇◇

25 SEPTEMBER 2013

Five element acupuncture on the move in China

I am delighted that plans are well advanced for Mei and Guy to go Nanning again in November, and however sad I am that I can't accompany them this time I am so happy that these two former students of mine are continuing with my work over there. One of my worries has been that my recent illness has made it impossible to give the regular support for our students in China that they need to strengthen their five element understanding, so that a visit from Mei and Guy takes some of this burden from me.

We still receive encouraging news about our students' continuing progress over there, and, as evidence of this, I give below a lovely email which Mei has just received from one of our students now practising five element acupuncture in Beijing.

She thanks Mei for her encouragement, and goes on to say:

'I have some good news to tell you; at the beginning the people in charge of our clinic didn't allow me to practise 5EA, so they only let me treat those patients who couldn't be helped by other means (herbs or TCM acupuncture). After two months, they saw how amazingly 5EA worked. Then I was allowed to practise 5EA. On top of that, they start charging much more for 5EA than other acupuncture. And very often they hand me the difficult and complicated cases. This is, on the one hand, stressful to me, being so young and inexperienced; on the other hand, I think people start to recognize and accept 5EA since it has proved its beauty.'

I'm so glad that five element acupuncture is now recognized as helping 'difficult and complicated cases', and is even being charged at a higher rate, presumably because it is seen as offering a better quality of acupuncture!

◇◇◇◇◇◇◇◇◇

10 OCTOBER 2013
What's in a name?

I have often been asked why I call a person's element their guardian element. And my answer to this is always the same. When I first learned about the elements and each person's attachment to one element, we called that element the person's CF, an abbreviation for the Causative Factor of Disease, coined by JR Worsley. During my years of study under him it was clear that he regarded the CF not simply as the cause of disease, the place of weakness in the five element circle where illness might strike, but as the focal point for a person's life, both as regards ill-health and health. In other words, this element was just as much the causative factor of good health as of disease.

I like to move away from the emphasis on disease implied by the term CF to a wider and more positive interpretation, and coined the phrase guardian element, because that is how I see the element we are endowed with in its widest sense. When weak it may well cause illness, but when strong it defends us, sheltering us under its wings, like some guardian angel watching over us – hence the term.

But whether we call an element our CF, our guardian element or, another phrase often used, our constitutional element, matters not one jot, provided that we recognize that our individual character is shaped, body and soul, by that element's features. So you can take your pick.

◇◇◇◇◇◇◇◇◇

17 OCTOBER 2013

How important is it that that a five element practitioner is sure of their own element?

One of the problems I face now when teaching students about five element acupuncture is that they are all too often unsure of their own element, and this casts a shadow of insecurity over their belief in five element practice as a whole. I think that this has a lot to do with there being so few five element teachers around now confident enough to make a diagnosis (see my blog of 11 September 2013), plus the understandable reluctance of even experienced practitioners to venture a diagnosis in case they step on the toes of a colleague who may be treating the student. So there is now greater timidity about moving into the area of diagnosing than there was in the good old days when we all clamoured to have JR Worsley diagnose us with the heartfelt approval of whatever practitioner we happened to have at the time.

Gone are those days and with them is gone the certainty which this led to. As I have often said, our particular guardian element shapes the whole of our life, including how we interact with our patients. Not to understand the nature of that interaction is to lose much essential information about our patients and may also cloud our judgement. It can certainly undermine our faith in what we are doing.

So I plead with all those who practise or are studying five element acupuncture to persist in their efforts to work out what their own element is, and, if they feel their treatment is not supporting them in the way they hoped, to dare discuss this with their practitioner. A practitioner must always listen if a patient, particularly another practitioner, is unhappy with the treatment offered. As everybody knows, it will always take some time to find the right element, and all of us five element practitioners should welcome any input from our colleagues to help us in any way reach a correct diagnosis, rather than, as is all too likely, feeling threatened.

If a practitioner is unsure of their own element, how effective do we think the treatments they offer others will be, based as they will be on an underlying feeling of insecurity?

◇◇◇◇◇◇◇◇◇

20 OCTOBER 2013

Mixing business with pleasure: an example of the Metal element, particularly for those in Australia

I was watching an Australian cricketer talking on TV, and wondered, as I always do, what element I thought he was. Suddenly I realized that his eyes reminded me of somebody. 'Who was it?', I thought, and gradually pinned it down to the eyes of that famous English actor, Laurence Olivier, who I had always thought of as definitely being Metal, particularly because of his voice. So was this cricketer Metal, too? Luckily the interview was quite a long one and I had plenty of time to watch and listen to him carefully. And yes, I decided to diagnose him as Metal, a preliminary diagnosis, of course, which was only my first hypothesis, but one that I felt as happy with as I could be after only ten minutes listening to him and watching his interaction with his interviewer.

His eyes were definitely sad, and had that far-away, serious look I associate with Metal. And the way he talked, too, was familiar to me as pointing me towards some of the Metal people I know. He spoke carefully, as if he had been working through things very systematically, and he was keen to answer the interviewer's questions in as clear and straightforward a way as possible. There was no attempt to try to engage the interviewer in any kind of relationship, as Fire or Earth might have done. At the end of the interview I was left with a feeling of having been in the presence of somebody very self-contained. All of this pointed to the Metal element, I thought.

Of course you will have to be somebody as keen on cricket as those in India or Australia to track down any interviews with this particular cricketer, but for those who want to have a good example of Metal to add to their library of Metal characteristics look for anything about the Australian cricketer, Ryan Harris, that you can find. And, whilst you are doing that, if you want a good comparison with the Fire element, you can do no better than watching the Australian cricket captain, Michael Clarke, who is an excellent example of a contrasting approach to being interviewed.

I have always enjoyed watching sport since I was a little girl and we were taken by our father to see many of the events in the 1948 Olympic Games. Now I can enjoy this from an additional angle, not only from the point of view of the sport itself, but adding to it a bit of spice by trying to work out the athletes' elements. This makes my TV watching both an enjoyable and an instructive exercise. As the saying goes, it is a good way of mixing business with pleasure.

◇◇◇◇◇◇◇◇◇

28 OCTOBER 2013

You are the best acupuncture textbook you will ever read

Following on from my blog of 17 October 2013 about practitioners being sure of their element, there is another important reason for this. In our lifetime each of us will only get to understand one element out of the five deeply from inside as it were, that of our own guardian element – that is, unless we believe, as I do not, that we change elements during our lifetime. That being so, we need to use this insider knowledge to our advantage, by studying ourselves closely.

We think we know ourselves, but I have found that, even after 30 years of close study of myself and my element Fire, I can still surprise myself with my reactions to a situation. It is only when I look closely at a particular response of mine that I realize, often to my own amusement, how typical of the Small Intestine it is, and therefore how much new light I myself continue to shed on this aspect of Fire.

Of course, being the Small Intestine part of Fire, and therefore only too happy to sort everything which comes my way, it is inevitable that I will be particularly concerned with constantly analyzing my reactions in that endlessly busy way the Small Intestine, the 'sorter', always does, but there is a lesson here for practitioners of other elements. We are all walking textbooks teaching us in detail about one of the five elements. By knowing ourselves well, we will therefore gain a deep understanding of at least one-fifth of the five element circle.

So to help those of you who are not of the Fire element, but who would like to understand how Fire, and Inner Fire in particular, reacts to different situations, I will keep on doing what I have done in previous blogs, and give you insights into the busy workings of my Small Intestine. At the same time I will try not to neglect the other elements, but what I write about these will always be slightly coloured by my own element, and therefore be slightly from an outsider's point of view rather from the inside. Those of other elements will have to be their own textbooks for these.

Rather frivolously, I have been thinking how very convenient it would be if all five element acupuncturists could find four other practitioners, one from each of the remaining elements, so that together they can form the complete circle of the elements and give themselves the opportunity continuously to share their personal insights with each other.

◇◇◇◇◇◇◇◇◇

1 DECEMBER 2013
The elements as filters

I was doing some cooking a few days ago, and poured the cooked spaghetti through a sieve to drain it. As I was doing this, the thought came to me that each element, like my spaghetti, needs a filter through which life is sieved. I only have one kitchen sieve, but each element has its own, with its own particular mesh allowing only certain things through.

When our energies become unbalanced, some of these meshes become blocked and can no longer filter what they should. Viewed in this way, treatment for the energy blocks with which any five element practitioner is familiar, such as those for a Husband/Wife imbalance or Entry/Exit blocks, can be seen as shaking the sieve in different ways to allow it to filter what has been blocking it.

I think the concept of the elements as sieves with different-sized meshes is a further rather neat illustration to help me understand what I do.

◇◇◇◇◇◇◇◇◇

2 DECEMBER 2013
It's never too late…

I came across this quotation in a book I was reading. 'It's never too late to be what you ought to have been.' It was attributed to the writer, George Eliot.

I like this very much, and it chimes with some of the thoughts I have been having. We should all live our lives with the thought that today may be our last day, and, if it is, have we been, as George Eliot say, 'what we ought to have been'? So I am asking myself this question now.

When you have been ill, as I have been (though now thankfully well on the way to full recovery), it makes you re-assess the whole of your life. For example, the two cancelled trips to China forced me to look again at how I was going to implement my teaching programme there, and how often I would be travelling over there in the future. And the success of Mei and Guy's visit without me to shepherd them around has made me realize yet again the truth of the saying that none of us is indispensable.

One thing I must do is learn to leave behind those many regrets we all have for the things not done or done imperfectly (our Metal regrets). I cannot now undo what I have done imperfectly, but I can undo how I view what I have done. And I think this is the secret of 'being who we ought to have been'. One of the greatest lessons our life must teach us is that we must learn to accept that at any point in that life we could only do what we could cope with doing. It's all too easy for other people, looking at us from the outside, to think we could or should have done things differently. We could not, because at that time that is all we could do. To accept our imperfections in this way is a necessary lesson to learn, and, once learnt, will surely help us a little further on the way to being 'what we ought to have been'.

◇◇◇◇◇◇◇◇

10 DECEMBER 2013
Don't ask our patients to reassure us!

We can so easily fall into the habit of asking for confirmation from our patients that our treatment is helping them. It is not our patients' job to make us feel better; it is ours to make them feel better. So we should avoid asking a question like, 'How are you feeling now?' at the end of treatment, because this is usually our way of asking for reassurance.

This is why it is important to remember the following:

It takes times for treatment to percolate through, so we should not expect patients to feel an immediate effect. It may take some days before patients are aware of any change.

Some people are not sufficiently self-aware to register that things have actually improved. This may be for several reasons. They may be reluctant to trust that things can get better, or uncertain whether things won't just go back to being how they were. They may also be unwilling to admit to any improvement for fear that we may start losing interest in continuing to see them.

'Feeling better' is a very subjective assessment of how we feel. As energy starts to return to greater balance, there may be all kinds of reactions as patients get used to adjusting to the changes inside them. There is often an unsettling time as patients have to learn to cope with what may be strange new feelings.

The only things we as practitioners should learn to rely upon are our own observations of change (or no change). We should look carefully at our patients as they leave at the end of treatment to see whether they look any different. And these changes will always be very subtle, a slightly brighter look in the eye, a brisker way of walking, a slightly warmer smile.

I was reminded of this yesterday after I had treated an Earth patient of mine, who came in looking worried and rather depressed, and left looking as if his spirit had received a welcome uplift. I felt that the person walking out of the door was quite different to the one who came in. He himself said as he left, without any prompting from me, 'I feel much better now.' This was an unexpected bonus for me, and left me feeling, yet again, what a lovely, yet profoundly simple calling is five element acupuncture.

For those interested to know what treatment I gave, it was: GV 14 (Great Hammer) (3 moxas), AEPs (back shu points) of Stomach and Spleen, III (Bl) 20, 21 (7 moxas), followed by the source points of Stomach and Spleen, XI (St) 42, XII (Sp) 3 (3 moxas). When he came in, he looked so resigned in a passive kind of a way that I thought his Earth element could benefit from being given a boost from GV (DM) 14, Great Hammer, before I did the AEPs.

14 DECEMBER 2013

It's all right to change your mind about a person's guardian element

One of the people who came to our seminar last week pointed out that I had changed my mind about Nigella Lawson's element. I had shown them a newspaper photo which, I told them, clearly showed the frightened eyes of a Water person. I was reminded that apparently I had included her as an example of Earth in one of my earlier lists of famous people.

I always emphasize how difficult it is to pinpoint a person's element, particularly that of a famous person whom I only know from the TV. Perhaps, indeed, it is a bit risky of me to make the selections that I do, because I can so obviously only too easily get things wrong. But somebody has to have the courage to stick their neck out, otherwise novice practitioners would have few examples of the elements to base their understanding on. I therefore do the best I can, however inadequately I may sometimes be doing this. My justification here is that I now have 30 years' experience to draw upon, whilst students have none at all, and as I always tell everybody, we owe those coming after us to hand on whatever knowledge we have acquired.

I hope that most of the examples I give, such as those of David Beckham and Elvis Presley in my *Keepers of the Soul*, are still valid, but if those reading what I write disagree with me, that is all to the good, because it forces them to study the elements deeply and develop their own understanding. And in any case, until I treat a person, I am never sure that I have found the right element.

I think, therefore, that I need to continue doing this, otherwise there would be so few examples to offer those who are unfamiliar with the elements. It is also good that I offer myself as a living example of somebody who doesn't mind getting things wrong and admitting to it. As I have said on many occasions, we all need to be humble enough in whatever field we work to accept that we will get things wrong, and to have the courage to admit that we have. Perhaps the next time I see Nigella Lawson on TV I may change my mind yet again, and opt for another element. It should not matter if I do. And will I mind? No. After all, to err is human…

◇◇◇◇◇◇◇◇◇

20 DECEMBER 2013
The symbolism of symptoms

It is always important to consider where physical symptoms appear on the body, and the nature of these symptoms. If we think of the body as housing our soul, as we should as acupuncturists for whom body and soul are one, then a symptom of the body must bear a close relationship to the soul encased within this body. I was reminded of this recently when helping a fellow practitioner with one of her patients who had been suffering for six years from a debilitating condition which affected her throat. Not only did this make speech difficult, but it gave her the constant feeling of being throttled. She had had all kinds of treatment, but nothing had so far helped.

When questioned about whether anything had happened at the time this started six years ago, it turned out that this was when a very much loved father-in-law had suddenly died.

This man had been very loving and caring, all that her own father, dead many years ago, had not been. The mention of her father-in-law made me wonder what her relationship to her own father was which had caused her husband's father to play such a prominent role in her life. I could see that any mention of her own father caused her a great deal of stress, so probing gently a little more I discovered that he had abused her sexually when she was a teenager, something she had told nobody until now. Without distorting the facts and the timescale in any way, it was not too fanciful to interpret the loss of her beloved father-in-law as an event which re-awakened the trauma of her abuse by her father and therefore proved the catalyst for the appearance of her throat problems. It is likely that her father threatened her if she told anybody about the abuse, consigning her to enforced silence, in effect a form of suffocation. This could be regarded as a possible cause for the appearance of the physical symptom of a throttled voice.

Apart from work on her element (Earth), I suggested that we add a point which I like very much, CV (RM) 22, the Window of Conception Vessel. I feel it allows light to shine upon this most important central pathway, and, in her case, was exactly located where she experienced the feelings of suffocation. I will find out in the coming weeks whether this first admission of the abuse she suffered and the treatment we gave her have helped her fully regain her voice. As she left, her practitioner told me that her voice already sounded stronger and more normal.

I think the two thoughts in my final blog below bring this book to an appropriate full stop. Certainly in looking back over the four years in which I have been writing these blogs, I would like to feel that I have indeed forgiven myself for what I may have done wrong, and altered my approach to the past.

20 DECEMBER 2013
Two thoughts

Maturity is accepting that we have done the best we could and forgiving ourselves for what we now see we have done wrong.

We can't alter the past, but we can alter our approach to the past.

CONCLUSION

I have had to re-read all of my blogs several times to see which are worth preserving within the permanent covers of a printed book rather than in their more ephemeral blog form stored on a computer. I have gained a surprising amount from this exercise of tailoring them into the shape of a book, having very much enjoyed re-acquainting myself with my thoughts, almost as though they were new to me. It is interesting how thoughts which have gestated within me, have been created in my mind and written down by my pen, somehow change their character once they are on the written page, escaping from my clutches and taking on an independent life. This appears to me to be much truer of thoughts preserved in book form than in those written with a blog in mind.

So drawing my blogs together into this book has been a surprisingly pleasurable time for me in which I got to know a part of myself again that I had almost, but not quite, forgotten.